FROM
ALLERGIES
TO HEALTH

T0204651

FROM ALLERGIES TO HEALTH

MANAGING A PLANT-BASED DIET
TO TAKE CONTROL OF YOUR HEALTH

ELLEN WAX

TOTTEN
POND
PRESS

A NOTE TO THE READER

This book is designed to provide helpful information on the subjects discussed. It is not meant to be used to diagnose or treat any medical condition. For diagnosis or treatment of a medical problem, consult your physician, especially regarding symptoms that may require medical attention. Readers with a medical condition should seek professional advice before changing their dietary or exercise plan.

FROM ALLERGIES TO HEALTH
by Ellen Wax

© 2019 by Ellen Wax
Published by Totten Pond Press
Brookline, MA 02446
info@tottenpondpress.com
All rights reserved.
No part of this book may be reproduced or transmitted in any form or by any means without the written permission of the publisher.

ISBN 978-1-7332628-0-4
Printed in Canada

Cover and interior design by Susan Livingston

Photography credits
Cover photo collage: © Romastudio | Dreamstime.com (main image, apple), © Jolanta Dabrowska | Dreamstime.com (blueberry), © Onepony | Dreamstime.com (kale), bergamont/Shutterstock.com (bok choy), © Fascinadora | Dreamstime.com (broccoli); Back cover: MasterQ/Shutterstock.com

Nattika/Shutterstock.com (page 5), learesphoto/Shutterstock.com (page 6), S.nilapan/Shutterstock.com (page 15), © Thodonal | Dreamstime.com (page 16), © Fortyforks | Dreamstime.com (page 80), © Sharona Jacobs (page 152)

To Rika Cohen, my friend and
Alexander Technique teacher,
who saw what I didn't see
and encouraged me
to solve my allergy problems
with the plant-based diet
that changed my life.

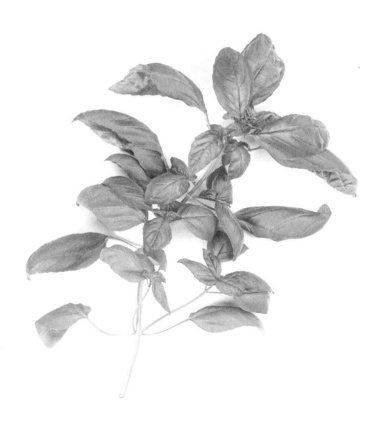

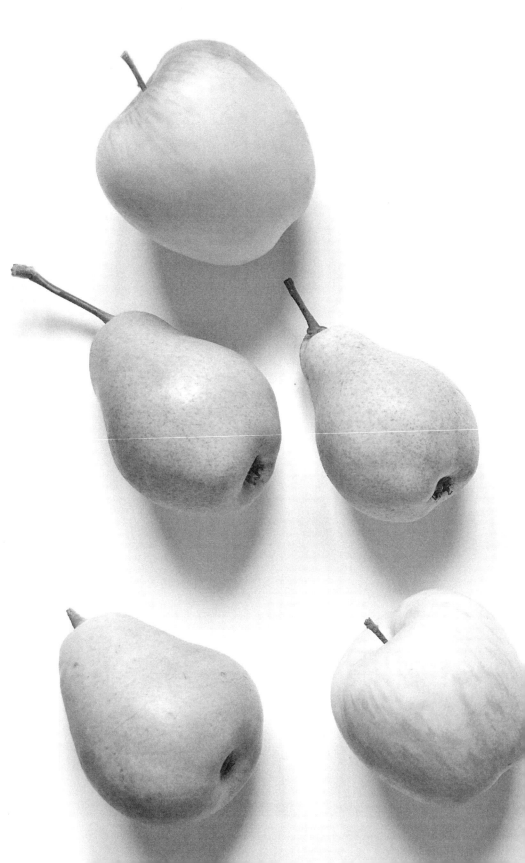

CONTENTS

PREFACE

From Allergies to Health describes how I overcame lifelong allergies by adopting a primarily plant-based diet and making other healthy lifestyle changes. This experience proved to be life-changing. I not only overcame my allergy problems but also learned about the power of food—about how what we eat, the way we eat, and when we eat can affect both health and mood.

After changing my approach to food and physical activity, I no longer was bothered by allergies and I lost unwanted weight. I've sustained these changes for over twenty years by connecting my diet and wellness activities with the planning and project management techniques I used professionally as a Director of Computer Systems Technology.

The idea for this book grew out of the many conversations I've had with people who want to take more control of their health and the realization that my method can be applied to a range of health concerns.

The first step toward my long-term success was education. Education helped me know where to begin and how to proceed. From classes, books, and experts I learned about:

- the relationship between diet and health
- diet and lifestyle practices that support good health
- menu-planning, cooking, and other aspects of a plant-based diet
- interpreting and responding to visual and other health markers

Going from the classroom to actually making the dietary and lifestyle changes was a challenge. Figuring out how to sustain these changes was even more challenging. In the following pages, you'll read about my journey from allergies to health, including my allergy background, the diet and lifestyle practices that changed my life, and the planning and project management techniques I've used to remain virtually allergy-free since the 1990s.

My great-aunt Sadie was an enthusiastic supporter of my new diet and enjoyed the meals I prepared. Plant-based food was always an important part of her family's meals and I remember grocery shopping with her when I was young. We would travel to several stores before she found the variety of fresh vegetables and fruit she sought. As we wished each other a Happy New Year in her 98th year she announced: "If you're healthy, you're happy."

Aunt Sadie had moved to an assisted living facility the previous year and immediately embraced the people she met and the activities there. She never lost her interest in her old and new families, in how she conducted her life, or in her health. She aged gracefully with her mental abilities intact until she passed away at the age of 107.

INTRODUCTION

"*You* gave up eating meat?" my cousin exclaimed at a family dinner. He couldn't believe it—he knew I had been a regular customer at his local butcher shop. I was astounded myself. But things change and we change. With chronic health problems, especially, what works for us one day may not work the next, or something we're doing no longer matches what we need. When we look for solutions and don't find them, we tend to move on, accepting what we believe we can't change. Yet, as I discovered, if we remain open to possibilities, a solution may find us.

I had seasonal and other allergies as far back as I can remember, and they persisted despite many attempts to find a solution or reduce their symptoms. My choice of remedies was limited to avoidance, which wasn't always possible, or medication that worked only somewhat and had side effects. Because I could not find a good alternative, I lived with all the sneezing and other debilitating allergy symptoms that had become a part of me.

Then several things happened that encouraged me to solve my allergy problems:

- My symptoms worsened.
- A friend urged me to try a plant-based diet for my allergies and recommended I attend a one-week residential course to learn to cook plant-based food.
- I went to the course, and by the end of the week I realized I felt much better.

While listening to a presentation about the relationship between diet and allergies, I had an "aha moment" in which I suddenly realized that my allergies might be a solvable problem instead of the permanent feature they had become in my life. Equipped with new information about the effect diet can have on allergies, an introduction to cooking plant-based food, and examples of an organized approach to implementing a plant-based diet, I realized I could apply planning and project management techniques I used every day at work to manage a new diet. I wanted to fix my allergy problems the way I fixed computer problems at work.

I have a considerable amount of experience solving problems from my background in math and from working with mainframe computer systems.[1] After college, I began working as a computer programmer for the Raytheon Company. For several years I worked on a project to build a global simulation model. When the project ended, I went to work as a systems program-

---

1 Mainframes, which were the first computer systems, now are used primarily by large organizations for critical applications where a failure or downtime is costly or catastrophic. They are also used for applications with very large data requirements, such as census data, or those with very high usage requirements, such as transaction processing.

mer at MIT but left a year later to join Interactive Data, a computer company that provided online access to historical financial data and closing stock market prices to large financial and other institutions. At Interactive Data, I designed and programmed operating system software for the mainframes that hosted the online service. Careful planning and implementation were necessary to meet the security, reliability, and availability goals of the service. Accomplishing these goals was not only challenging but gave me the opportunity to hone my systems development and management skills. I stayed with Interactive Data for over thirty years as it grew from forty people to over a thousand. During that time, in addition to computer systems design and programming, I was involved with many aspects of management.

I hadn't spent a lot of time in my kitchen, but I did have a lot of project management experience in which education, accuracy, and efficiency were critical to success. I believed that by approaching a new diet as a project, I could manage my way to succeeding with it. Treating the diet as a project also helped me incorporate it into my life. I knew the additional planning, shopping, and cooking would be easier and more enjoyable if I could do it efficiently. Moreover, by taking a management approach, I wasn't relying *only* on self-discipline to follow through with the diet. I knew from past experience with weight-loss diets that that method hadn't work for me.

After adopting a plant-based diet and becoming more physically active, I achieved what I, at one time, thought was impossible. I was free of allergy symptoms. At the same time, I lost excess weight. I expected to miss my former favorite foods, such as ice cream and pizza, but found I didn't. I felt healthier and happier eating the food on my new diet.

As an unexpected bonus, I learned how to manage my health better. I could do something my doctors couldn't—I could monitor my allergies and overall health on a day-to-day basis just as I managed my computer systems, which I monitored daily in order to forestall problems. Similarly, by paying attention to how I felt, I could adjust my diet to avoid problems. I've continued to rely on medical and health professionals for health care, but I successfully manage my allergies on my own without medication.

With today's increased awareness of the interaction between diet and health, specialized diets are more likely to be used as part of a healthy lifestyle and to address problems such as allergies. In addition to macrobiotic, vegan, and vegetarian, these include gluten-free, acid-alkaline, and a number of others. I can apply what I've learned from changing my diet to exploring any of these. It has given me experience with making dietary changes that I can build on as I learn more and as things change.

As you read this book, try making the changes that appeal to you or that seem manageable. Whether you make one change or many, you too may be surprised to find that they help you feel healthier and happier.

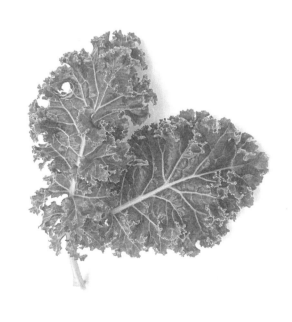

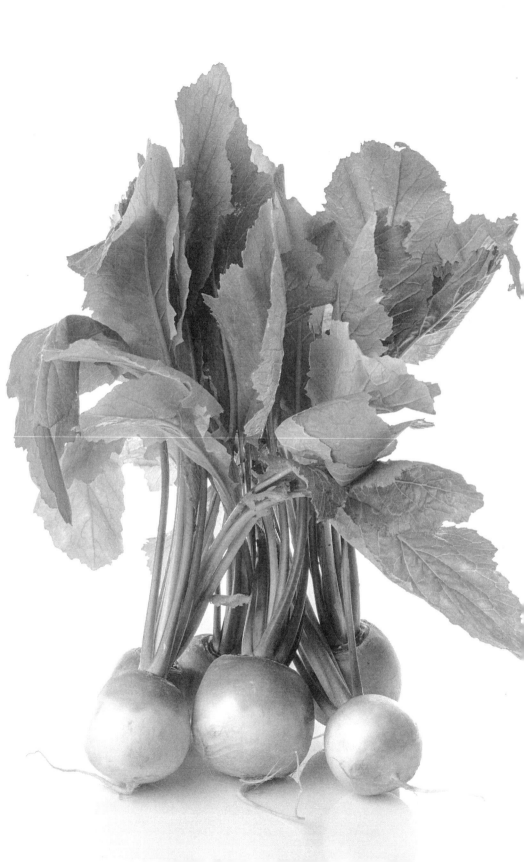

PART 1

ALLERGIES AND OVERCOMING THEM

CHAPTER 1
ALLERGIES

Allergies are sneaky—one minute you're feeling fine and the next you're miserable. Allergies are considered to be the result of an overactive or hypersensitive immune system and unless provoked by the presence of an allergen, they remain invisible. When symptoms do appear, they can be mistaken for a cold, a headache, a skin rash, unexplained weight gain, or other health problem. Unless they cause anaphylaxis—a severe reaction—allergies generally are not life-threatening. Chronic allergies, however, *are* disruptive to good heath. For instance, the common symptoms of a stuffy nose and mouth breathing are not only uncomfortable but can lead to other health problems.[1]

Allergies also are complicated and they continue to puzzle

---

1 Note: Allergies that are severe enough to trigger anaphylaxis require medical supervision and are beyond the scope of this book.

the researchers who investigate such things as why some people have them and others don't.

MY ALLERGY BACKGROUND

Beginning in childhood I had multiple allergies with symptoms that often mimicked a cold. I also suffered with asthma until the age of 12. Looking back, I was exposed to many allergy triggers. We lived in an old house with a damp basement, and we had a variety of pets. Growing up in a close-knit family with excellent bakers, I ate delicious cookies, cakes, and other baked treats every day. At the time, we weren't aware that baked-flour products, especially those made with yeast, can be a problem for someone with allergies or that eating too much sugar can cause chronic inflammation that makes allergies worse.

Skin prick tests showed I had environmental allergies and was extremely allergic to cats. I had such a strong reaction when tested for cat allergies that I fainted from it. Shortly afterwards, my parents gave our cat away. The doctor prescribed allergy injections, but they didn't help. I continued to sneeze a lot, and until I no longer had asthma I avoided activities that provoked wheezing, such as riding my bicycle too far or running.

When allergy injections had no effect, my allergies became something I "lived with." Medication helped relieve my symptoms, but only somewhat. I was the kid who always was sneezing, and the adult who never left the house without a supply of tissues. I tried to avoid things I was allergic to, but some, like dust, mold, and pollen, are nearly impossible to avoid.

I live in New England, known for its colorful fall season. For me, though, fall meant ragweed pollen and hay fever, lots of sneezing, watery eyes, and feeling miserable. Springtime allergies hadn't been a problem for me until one year I began experiencing eye inflammation. Several years later, at times I developed a head rash from tree pollen if I walked under trees without wearing a hat.

Around the time my allergies worsened, my schedule had changed and I was dining out more. I also was gaining weight. I was away from home several evenings a week, and my dinner was late and often pizza, alternating with fast food burgers and healthier fish or chicken dinners. I kept gaining weight and my allergy symptoms got worse. I noticed that I sometimes experienced cold symptoms after eating pizza, but I didn't explore further than that. There seemed to be a correlation, but "sometimes" wasn't compelling enough for me to stop eating pizza completely.

Despite all the clues, I never connected the dots when it came to environmental allergies and food. I had checkups, tried new medications, avoided what I thought would cause problems, and lived with allergies.

Then, a friend urged me to try a plant-based diet to relieve my allergy symptoms. At the time, the connection between diet and allergies was not widely known, but she had had friends with allergies, who had done well on the diet.

I had been growing concerned because my allergies were getting worse, and the possibility of eliminating them intrigued me. If medication had worked well, I may not have looked further. But the medication that did help had side effects, which limited its usefulness.

I decided to follow my friend's recommendation and was introduced to a way of eating and lifestyle changes that dramatically reduced my allergy symptoms.

It was only after I started to become free of them that I realized how much they had bothered me. Whether it was the impact of the new diet on my allergies, other benefits of the diet, or a combination of both, I was more energetic, lost excess weight, and was happier. I noticed I was able to focus more easily at work. Even though I was spending more time shopping for food and cooking, I had more energy with which to do it. Life, in general, was easier.

The following chart shows the results of the IgE allergy tests[2] I had in 1989, 2003, and 2009. I was tested in 1989 because of worsening allergy symptoms and again in 2003 and 2009 to measure the changes.

The 2003 and 2009 results show the improvements from changing to a plant-based diet, which I began in 1994. To compare the tests, I used the qualitative interpretation of the results instead of the numeric values because in the intervening

---

2 IgE (Immunoglobulin E) tests are allergen-specific tests that are used to diagnose allergies. They measure the blood level of IgE antibodies produced when a person's immune system overreacts to the presence of an allergen, a substance that causes an allergic reaction.

years the method of IgE testing, which affects the numeric values, changed.

ALLERGEN-SPECIFIC IGE ALLERGY TEST RESULTS

ALLERGEN	DEC 1989	DEC 2003	SEPT 2009
RAGWEED	Very High	Low	Very Low
MOLD	Moderate	Low	Very Low
DUST	Moderate	Undetectable	Undetectable
CATS	Moderate	Undetectable	Undetectable

In 1989, I was highly allergic to ragweed and moderately allergic to mold, dust, and cats, although at the time I had a strong allergic reaction to some cats. The subsequent tests in 2003 and 2009 show a low or very low response to ragweed and mold with an undetectable response to dust and cats.

The results reflect my experience well. In 1989, I had a very high "tissue count"—I used a lot of them. Now, I'm relatively symptom-free. I've continued to avoid cats because at times I have a reaction to them, although one that's much less severe than it was before I changed my diet.

THE ESCALATING ALLERGY PROBLEM

The allergy landscape has changed dramatically. A significantly larger percentage of people have allergies, and the incidence of life-threatening allergies has created the need for warning signs in restaurants and on the packaging of food that is known to cause allergic reactions in some people.

Before placing your order please inform your server if a person in your party has a food allergy.

—Sign seen in restaurants

Allergies have increased globally, more so in the West. Recently, I spoke with someone who moved from Southeast Asia to New England six years ago. She told me that for the past two years her eyes have become irritated during the spring from a pollen allergy and she has now declared herself "westernized."

Fueled by the growing problem, advances in both conventional medicine and alternative practices are leading to new strategies for dealing with allergies. Following a plant-based diet to control environmental allergies was a new idea when I began. Today, however, both environmental and food allergies are far more prevalent, and plant-based diets are used more often to treat them.

THE MICROBIOME AND ALLERGIES

Emerging knowledge about the human microbiome and the microbes in our gut and elsewhere on our bodies represents a leap forward in understanding how we humans are organized. The microbiome has been described as a second genome that, unlike the human genome, is directly influenced by changes in diet and other factors, such as antibiotic use, exercise, and sleep. Thus, the microbiome is different from DNA—a person's genetic makeup—which is unchangeable. While genes may predispose someone to a disease, whether or not genes are expressed—or activated—often depends on a number of factors that, like the microbiome, include diet, environment, lifestyle, and stress.

Researchers have discovered that the microbes in the microbiome are essential for our development, immunity, and nutrition, and that starting from the moment we're born, all aspects of our health, including our immune system and allergies, are influenced by our environment and our diet. Studies show a relationship between genes and the microbiome—genes influence the microbiome and the microbiome can influence whether or not genes are expressed.

I first learned about the microbiome from *The Good Gut*, a highly informative book that presents information that medical research is bringing to light about the microbiome and how it affects our overall health and well-being. The authors describe how we can use the information that's available now to adjust our diet to support our microbiome. They discuss such topics as the importance of dietary fiber and fermented foods and the problems caused by antibiotics, all of which alter the gut microbiome.

Knowledge of the microbiome expanded in 2008 with the Human Microbiome Project, and since then the microbiome has attracted a lot of interest within the scientific community and among the public. In June 2017, the American Museum of Natural History in New York opened the exhibit "Inside You," which is about the microbiome. It includes information from *The Good Gut* and other sources.

Much remains unanswered, but researchers are continuing to unravel the secrets of the microbiome. While there's no comparison in terms of the complexity of the human body, the discussion about the microbiome reminded me of the early days of the computer operating system I worked on. At times it seemed to take on a life of its own, exhibiting behavior that wasn't predicted. Often this happened because the developers hadn't anticipated how the system would be used.

When these problems occurred, however, they were relatively easy to fix by modifying code or by adding hardware. It may be too early to know if we can look forward to a day when we can identify and fix dysfunctions in our microbiome as easily or whether the microbiome will remain too complex and reactive to its environment for that to be a possibility.

CHAPTER 2
DIET AND HEALTH

EDUCATION

Plant-based diets are more common in the United States today, but they were relatively rare in 1994 when a friend urged me to try one to help my allergies. Whether it was my worsening allergies or good timing, I listened. She knew people with allergies who had had success with a macrobiotic plant-based diet and thought it could relieve my allergy symptoms. Having spoken with them about their experiences, my friend stressed the importance of knowing how to cook plant-based food in order to follow the diet well as she gave me the brochure for a weeklong program of cooking classes at the Kushi Institute. I was skeptical that changing my diet could make much of a difference, and although I liked vegetables, I questioned whether I was prepared to give up meat, cheese, and other food I liked. Despite my reservations, learning to cook all the grains and vegetables

I bypassed in grocery stores because I didn't know how to cook with them tipped the balance in favor of going to the program.

Once there, I found the first few days difficult. I enjoyed the classes; I didn't like the food. I wasn't familiar with pungent vegetables such as turnip and daikon radish, and I wondered about the seemingly inverse relationship between food that was good for me and food that smelled and tasted good.

Then things improved. I became more accustomed to the smells and tastes and enjoyed learning the language of vegetables—leafy green, round, root—and various ways to cook them. I had never been to a cooking class, and watching the instructors was fascinating as they skillfully demonstrated how to prepare and cook grains, beans, and vegetables. While cooking, they provided useful information, such as how to make grains and beans more digestible by soaking them overnight and the benefit of combining beans with kombu, a sea vegetable also known as kelp.

In addition to cooking classes, the instructors covered a wide range of topics related to health and macrobiotics. These included a discussion of the book *Standard Macrobiotic Diet*, macrobiotic philosophy, visual diagnosis, movement techniques, and lifestyle practices, such as chewing well. Taken together, the classes provided a multifaceted approach to improving health.[1]

---

1 The bibliography includes *Standard Macrobiotic Diet* and books about macrobiotic philosophy and related topics. Although *Standard Macrobiotic Diet* is out of print, used copies are available. A similar list of foods can be found in *The Complete Macrobiotic Diet*.

In a class about the effects of eating various foods, the instructor talked about the relationship between allergies and foods that tend to produce mucus, such as dairy products. He also revealed that as we began this new diet we might discover evidence that our body was eliminating excess from our old diet. As an example, he said that people who ate a lot of dairy foods and were starting a macrobiotic diet, which doesn't include dairy, might temporarily develop white patches on their arms from eliminating it.[2]

At the end of the week, as people were preparing to leave, a woman who had travelled from Denmark showed us several white patches on her arms that had appeared overnight—just as the instructor had described might happen to someone who had eaten a lot of dairy foods. I was already considering trying the macrobiotic diet, but when I saw the white patches, I was hooked. Witnessing the evidence of a detox process suggested to me that dietary changes might also eliminate residual effects of food I had eaten in the past. I was convinced that what I had learned could help with my allergies.

As further encouragement, I felt more energetic and hadn't needed the allergy medication I'd brought with me. I thought: I'm becoming accustomed to the food, and the allergies I've had all my life are a nuisance and getting worse. If changing my diet can make a difference, I'll try it.

---

2 Subsequently, I learned the elimination (detox) process is not as straightforward as it seemed when I first learned about it. It depends on a person's metabolism, the interaction between what someone is eating now and what they ate in the past, and other factors.

NEXT STEPS TO A NEW DIET

I returned home from the cooking classes excited to start my new diet and solve my allergy problems. I was expecting a lot from the diet and I knew it was up to me to give it a chance to succeed.

But the reality was daunting—food was such an important part of my life and relationships. I knew there would be ramifications to my lifestyle from starting a diet that was unusual, not to mention one that required more work, although I didn't know what their extent would be. More than likely, I thought, I wouldn't be joining friends on Saturday mornings for a leisurely breakfast of coffee and croissants or entertaining on the spur of the moment by going to my local market for cheese and crackers, chicken breasts, baking potatoes, frozen vegetables, dessert, and a log for the fireplace.

The week of classes had motivated me enough to overcome these doubts, however, and set the stage for the approach I took. I realized I would need to be more organized about eating. I was organized at work, but my eating tended to be chaotic. At various times, I had tried new diets that I thought were healthier or might help me lose weight, but they didn't last long, especially when they interfered with my social eating. If my new diet worked and I focused only on the food, I knew I might be tempted to go off it as soon as I started feeling better, just as I had with weight-loss diets. I needed a different strategy. As I describe in Chapter 3, Management and Problem-

Solving Techniques, I turned to the management tools I used every day at work to help me stay on the diet and integrate it into my life.

The classes had reminded me of work projects that began with education, and I began to think of my diet as a pilot project or experiment. To get started, I first had to organize my kitchen and concentrate on menu planning, shopping, and cooking.

After the classes ended, I had another week of vacation and took several days to plan my initial approach, organize my kitchen, and shop for food and kitchenware. While doing that, I cooked simple plant-based meals, such as brown rice, kale, and lentil soup.

MENU PLANNING

My guidelines for menu planning were:

- Plan meals around whole grains and grain products along with a variety of vegetables, beans, fruit, and other plant-based food
- Vary ingredients and cooking styles
- Avoid refined sugar and limit other natural sweeteners
- Avoid highly processed food
- Be mindful of the season and weather

I would be cooking plant-based food using macrobiotic recipes, bringing leftovers from dinner to work for lunch, and eating fish twice a week either at home or when dining out.

I knew my schedule would present a challenge—on weekdays I was away from home for ten hours or more, which included commuting two hours. But, I hadn't considered the implications of bringing lunch to work instead of conveniently buying it in the company cafeteria. Sitting down to plan menus, I realized that, for me, lunch was pivotal to the success of the entire experiment. If I didn't bring a satisfying lunch to work—no matter what else I did—I wouldn't stay on the new diet. I'd be tempted to buy food that wasn't part of the diet from the cafeteria and vending machines. This meant cooking dinner most nights to have the food I needed for lunch. It also meant eating breakfast and bringing healthy snacks so I wouldn't be overly hungry at lunchtime and tempted to supplement my lunch with fries or other cafeteria food.

With my schedule in mind and using a menu-planning format similar to the one on pages 94–95 in Chapter 7, I planned a week of menus guided by recipes from the cooking classes. The classes had emphasized eating good-quality organic food and varying ingredients and cooking styles to keep meals balanced, nutritious, and satisfying. My goal was to plan meals that followed their guidelines and that I would enjoy. The outline of each day's plan was similar:

Breakfast

Grain porridge
Steamed or quick-boiled leafy greens and other
    vegetables
Tea

Lunch

Leftovers from dinner that might include:

A grain or noodle dish

A vegetable dish

Soup or a bean dish

Pickles (some days)

Dessert (some days)

Snacks

Nuts, seeds, raw vegetables

Dinner

Soup

A grain or a noodle dish

A short-cooked vegetable dish (typically under
5 minutes)

A long-cooked vegetable dish (typically 20 minutes
or longer)

A bean dish (unless I was making a bean soup), a dish
made with a soy product such as tempeh, or fish

Pickles (some days)

Dessert (some days)

When making food selections, I used the recommendations in *Standard Macrobiotic Diet*, which classifies grains, vegetables, and beans as either for:

- Everyday use
- Occasional use (two or three times a week)
- To be used sparingly or avoided

For example: the everyday-use list for grains includes short-grain brown rice, medium-grain brown rice, millet, pearl barley, hulled barley, whole oats, buckwheat, and rye.

The food I'd no longer be eating included:

- All dairy products. Giving up cheese, pizza, yogurt, and ice cream would be more difficult than giving up milk. I only used it in my morning cereal, and I would now be substituting a healthier alternative because the cereal was processed and contained sugar.
- Poultry and meat. This eliminated chicken, steak, burgers, corned beef, hot dogs, and other meat products.

Among the food I'd eat much less of, if at all, were:

- Fries, chips, and other highly processed food.
- Yeasted bread, cakes, cookies, and other baked-flour goods.
- Desserts made with refined sugar. Instead, I'd be eating berries or lightly cooked tree fruit and puddings made with fruit, apple juice, and thickeners, such as agar flakes or kuzu root.

Sugar, Salt, and Oil

Sugar, salt, and oil are important components of any diet. Too much sugar, poor quality salt or oil, and too much or too little salt or oil all can undermine efforts to achieve good health through diet.

- Apple juice, rice syrup, barley malt, and maple syrup were recommended as alternative sweeteners in limited amounts depending on one's tolerance for sugar. Someone who has a low tolerance often can satisfy a desire for something sweet with sweet vegetables, such as carrots or squash.
- Good-quality sea salt was recommended for cooking instead of table salt. See Resources. Salt is not added to food after cooking, but a salty flavor is added with condiments such as gomashio, a sesame salt made by grinding roasted sesame seeds together with salt, shiso leaf powder, and umeboshi vinegar. Coming from a meat-based diet, I tended to use more salt than I needed and, over time, used less.
- Organic olive oil and sesame oil were recommended for everyday use.

SETTING UP A PLANT-BASED KITCHEN

My work schedule also influenced how I organized my kitchen. I needed to be efficient, and a well-organized kitchen saves time and makes cooking more enjoyable. As a first step, I eliminated the food I wouldn't be using and removed unnecessary kitchen items to make space for new kitchenware.

Food Staples

- **Grains:** several kinds of brown rice, including short-grain, medium-grain, sweet brown, brown basmati, and white basmati, millet, pearl barley, whole oats, and couscous

- **Pasta:** udon noodles, soba noodles, and other whole wheat pasta. Now I also use brown rice and other kinds of pasta.
- **Beans:** adzuki, black turtle, kidney, lentils, black soybeans, and chickpeas
- **Sea Vegetables:** nori, arame, dulse, kombu (kelp), and wakame
- **Nuts and Seeds:** almonds, walnuts, and pumpkin seeds
- **Condiments:** sea salt, naturally fermented shoyu, umeboshi plums, umeboshi vinegar, brown rice vinegar, and shiso powder. At first, I obtained these by mail order but now those that aren't available locally can be ordered online. See Resources.
- **Other:** barley miso, chickpea miso, unyeasted whole wheat bread made with sourdough starter, naturally fermented sauerkraut, sesame seeds, tahini, ginger, dried shitake mushrooms.

Kitchenware

I had pots, pans, and other basic kitchenware and added the following:

- **Jars** for storing grains, beans, and other food. Mason jars work well for this purpose.
- **Vegetable knives.** The most important addition to my kitchen was a good-quality vegetable knife. These knives simplify the tasks of cutting, slicing, mincing, and dicing and when used correctly are safer than a standard utility knife. Watching the cooks in my classes use a 7-inch Japanese Nakiri knife, a sharp

knife with a wide rectangular blade, I saw how effective it was. Another popular Japanese vegetable knife is the Santoku. Online instructional videos show how to use these and other vegetable knives. I use a Nakiri vegetable knife for most tasks, alternating occasionally with a small paring knife.

- **Chef's knife.** I often use a heavier chef's knife for cutting hard winter squash.
- **Cutting boards.** I use both wooden and bamboo cutting boards, which I wipe clean and let dry after each use. Bamboo is easier to care for, but because it is harder than wood, it dulls knives more quickly.
- **Fine mesh strainers and shallow stainless steel bowls.** Among other uses, these are useful for washing and soaking grains and beans. I use a flat, long-handled strainer to remove vegetables and other food from a pot or a steamer.
- **Sushi mats.** Bamboo sushi mats are used to roll sushi and also can be used as a cover when soaking or serving food.
- **Lunch bag, thermos food jars, and containers** for taking soups, stews, and other food to work for lunch.
- **Heavy pot with tight-fitting lid.** Some foods, especially beans and grains, benefit from cooking in a heavy pot with a tight-fitting lid, such as those made from enamel-coated cast iron.
- **Pressure cooker.** Pressure cookers are invaluable for cooking beans and some grains. Today's pressure cookers are improved and safer than the one we had years ago that exploded, sending the contents to the ceiling.

- **Cast-iron skillets.** These are inexpensive and a source of iron. They're good for occasional or frequent use depending on someone's tolerance for more iron in their diet.
- **Steamer pot.** A steamer pot, which is similar to a double boiler, is handy for steaming vegetables and warming food.
- **Stovetop heat diffuser/flame tamer.** A small, circular metal plate that when placed under a pot or pressure cooker helps to distribute heat evenly and prevent burning. I use a heat diffuser when cooking grains. They're available in most kitchenware shops and online.
- **Suribachi and surikogi.** Similar to a mortar and pestle, a Japanese suribachi is a grooved ceramic mortar used with a wooden surikogi. It's especially useful for making gomashio.
- **Medium-sized bowls** for soaking grains.
- **Wooden rice paddle, cooking chop sticks, long-handled wooden spoons.**
- **Ginger grater**
- **Covered glass bowls** for storing leftover food in the refrigerator.

SHOPPING

As far as I can tell, most projects—big or small—begin with shopping. Since I needed kitchenware, staples, and fresh food, my first stops were to a local kitchen shop that had a large assortment of glass jars and to a restaurant supply store.

Next I went to a Whole Foods market, which at the time

was called Bread and Circus. My list of vegetables included celery, leafy green vegetables (kale, collard greens, and mustard greens), round vegetables (broccoli, turnips, onions, and winter squash), and root vegetables (carrots, parsnips, and burdock). I was pleased to no longer be limited by lack of knowledge to lettuce, tomatoes, and a small number of other vegetables. Instead, I could choose from a seemingly endless, healthy-looking, colorful variety. Likewise, there were many more choices for grains and beans than were on my initial list.

FROM PLANNING TO PRACTICE

Now that my kitchen was transformed for plant-based cooking, I was ready to prepare three macrobiotic meals a day. All the classroom work, planning, and preparation paid off as I carefully followed recipes, soaked grains and beans, cut vegetables, made condiments, and cooked a variety of dishes.

The next step was preparing to bring lunch to work using my menu plan and new containers. I imagined what lunchtime would look like. I knew I wouldn't enjoy sitting at a table in the cafeteria surrounded by thermos bottles and small containers—nor would my lunch buddies. I decided I could easily plate my lunch. While people were buying lunch, I would transfer food from the containers and return them to my lunch bag.

Adjusting my schedule so I'd have time to cook was challenging. Mornings were manageable. I started earlier and became proficient at making breakfast and packing the lunch I prepared the night before. I found cooking dinner relaxing and enjoyable after a day at work and commuting. On days when

I wasn't home to cook dinner, I ate fish or plant-based-friendly food out and then prepared vegetarian sushi for lunch.

Still, I was finding it difficult to balance shopping for food and cooking with other activities. In order to be successful I had to cook meals with enough variety to be satisfying and to provide sufficient nutrition. Simple meals of sushi or lentil soup, brown rice, and kale were okay once in a while, but not on a regular basis.

Help arrived when I began attending Warren Kramer's cooking classes. Warren, an experienced cook and macrobiotic counselor, provided recipes and explained each step as he and his assistants cooked a complete dinner of soup, a grain dish, a bean dish, vegetable dishes, and dessert. Watching them prepare the meal, I learned more about cooking and how to be efficient in the kitchen. The classes also provided an opportunity to meet and exchange information with people who were eating a macrobiotic or other plant-based diet. Warren holds cooking classes in the Boston area and elsewhere. See Resources. If cooking classes aren't available in your area or if you can't travel to one, online classes can be helpful.

LIFESTYLE PRACTICES TO SUPPORT DIET AND HEALTH

Changing my diet without changing anything else would have reduced my allergy symptoms. Diet alone, however, very likely would not have eliminated them or resulted in my losing as much excess weight. In addition to my change in diet, I followed some of the macrobiotic-recommended lifestyle practices, such as regular mealtimes and walking outside daily, which have a beneficial synergistic effect with the diet.[3] At one time, these were part of everyday life, but with the faster pace of modern living, they have been forgotten or ignored.

EATING HABITS

Good eating habits are beneficial no matter what food we're eating. The macrobiotic recommendations related to eating habits reminded me of lessons I was taught during childhood. My family had regular mealtimes, and I was encouraged to eat without distractions, such as reading; to sit when eating; to eat slowly in order to chew food well; not to overeat; and not to eat before bedtime.[4] Our typical mealtimes—breakfast: 7 to 8 a.m., lunch: 12 p.m., and dinner: 6 to 7 p.m.—also coincided with macrobiotic recommendations for the healthiest eating times and for aligning with nature. They're based on the movement of the sun and are the same recommendations as in traditional Chinese medicine—breakfast: 7 to 9 a.m., lunch: 11 a.m. to 1 p.m., and dinner: 5 to 7 p.m.

Chew, Chew, Chew . . . chew. . . . Chewing is so important because digestion, aided by chewing, begins in the mouth. We can improve our digestion by chewing well. When I was intro-

---

3 Denny Waxman provides a comprehensive description of the lifestyle practices in *The Complete Macrobiotic Diet.*

4 I noticed that I slept better when I didn't lie down immediately after eating but allowed the recommended two to three hours before bedtime—something I now do routinely.

duced to macrobiotics, the guideline was to chew fifty times or more a mouthful, with one hundred times even better. Whether it's thirty times, fifty, or more, the importance of chewing thoroughly is undisputed. As I slowly chewed my way through meals, the more I chewed the better I felt, especially when eating fibrous foods such as brown rice. Some people naturally chew very well. I wasn't one of them, and paying attention to chewing helped me adapt to a high-fiber diet.

PHYSICAL ACTIVITY

The recommendations for physical activity include walking outside for thirty minutes a day; the body rub—gently rubbing the body with a hot, damp cotton washcloth once or twice a day; and staying active, whether with household chores such as cleaning and gardening, practices such as tai chi and yoga, or other activities.

I had considered myself fairly active, but I had never realized the positive impact doing something every day can have on one's health.

I began taking daily walks outside for thirty minutes or more unless it was unsafe for walking. At work, I walked around the office complex either after lunch or later in the afternoon, and I sometimes broke up the walk into two shorter walks. My afternoon walks were invaluable—they eliminated food cravings for something sweet and, if I had been struggling with a problem, they often helped to clarify my thinking.

The body rub took more time to get used to. I became a proponent of it after seeing friends transform their appearance from somewhat dull- and dry-skinned to fresh-looking after several months of doing the body rub.

SEASONAL EATING

Food that's grown locally is more nutritious, tastes better, and has the added benefit of supporting local farmers. Macrobiotic dietary guidelines are designed for a four-season temperate climate and recommend eating food that's grown in the same or similar climate zone.

Before modern communications and fast, low-cost transportation made it possible, the availability of food from other regions was limited. Now food from around the world is readily available throughout the year. This allows one to buy food, such as apples and kale, at times outside of the local growing season. It results, however, in fruits and vegetables that are grown in and are more suitable for the tropics finding their way to a table in a place with a four-season climate. Including this food in one's diet can have its drawbacks and lead to a dietary imbalance. Eating food that's compatible with one's local climate is healthier and also helps our bodies adjust to seasonal changes. For example, just as someone moving to New England from a tropical climate will adapt more easily to winter by bundling up, they also will feel better if they adjust their diet by limiting tropical fruit in favor of more hot drinks, hearty soups, and other foods that have a warming effect on the body. Paying attention to food grown locally or grown in a similar climate zone is a great way to start.

> Our appetites are the outcome of
> the foods we eat.
>
> —Antoine de Saint-Exupery

ADAPTING TO A PLANT-BASED DIET

As I expected, meal preparation—from menu planning to food shopping to cooking—required more time and effort than I was used to. I found, however, that I felt much better and had a lot more energy. Without question, it was a worthwhile tradeoff.

THE FIRST YEAR

Previously, my approach to eating had vacillated between eating what I considered a healthy western diet and what I referred to as "opportunistic eating." For example, when a gourmet bakery opened in my neighborhood, I began stopping for coffee and a croissant on my way to work, and when I was taking a class that began close to dinner time, I stopped nearby for a burger, fries, and hot chocolate.

Now, I was eating healthier food, preparing most meals at home, and becoming more adept at cooking. I continued going to cooking classes, which I found enjoyable and informative. We were served a delicious meal at the end of each class, letting us taste the recipes prepared by an expert cook.

With more experience, I noticed, for example, that after eating food that was salty or spicy, I craved something sweet, so

I began balancing tastes in a meal, often ending with a sweet vegetable. I also paid more attention to food choices, especially those on the "eat sparingly or avoid" list. These include night-shades, such as eggplant, white potatoes, tomatoes, and peppers that cause inflammation in some people. I eat few nightshades because there are many other choices. When the warm weather of August brings delicious, juicy tomatoes, though, I eat them in moderation.

Plant-based food is more likely to be served at parties and other events now, but in the beginning I often brought a dish to serve or a snack with me. When life got more complicated and I wasn't home as often to cook or when I was travelling, I brought food with me, took shortcuts, and otherwise kept as close to the diet and lifestyle habits as I could.

Having good alternatives made it easier to give up food I'd eaten all my life. I had always loved cheese and pizza. I expected to miss them, but I was surprised to find that I didn't. Six months after starting the diet, I tried some of my former favorites and discovered they no longer tasted as good as I remembered.

I experienced detox symptoms that can occur when making dietary changes, although nothing as dramatic as the white patches I describe earlier occurred. Had I not seen those and heard about the detox process in a class, however, I might have been more concerned when I developed flu-like symptoms with-out feeling like I had the flu, or when I had two bouts of laryn-gitis that each left me speechless for over a week and which no remedy helped. For a couple of years, I developed various skin rashes that came and went, and a small rash on the back of my neck that had bothered me for years before I began the diet occasionally got much worse. Two years later it was gone and hasn't returned.

At some point during the first year, I realized I wasn't returning to my former way of eating. I felt like a new person—lighter and with more energy. Although my allergy symptoms were not entirely gone at that point, they were so much better that I happily embraced this more orderly approach to diet and physical activity.

RELATIONSHIPS

Changing from a meat-based to a plant-based diet had a ripple effect on my relationships. It's an unavoidable consequence, and one that affects everyone differently depending on their health needs, family situation, and lifestyle. I wasn't quite sure what to expect.

Family

I hadn't anticipated the question my seven-year-old niece asked at a family meal when I brought some of my own food. She wondered why her family's food was good for her mother but not for me. Not having a ready answer, I mumbled something about allergies, but the experience made me realize that I needed to change my approach. Instead of bringing food only for myself, I brought rice dishes and vegetables that my family liked to share with them.

Friends

Whether or not they believed the diet would help, my friends knew I had allergy problems and understood why I was looking for a solution. Some friends liked my then-unusual, plant-based food while others supported what I was doing but weren't interested in eating the food. While I was learning how to cook my new recipes, I often supplemented meals with prepared food when I invited friends over.

I expected some resistance from my foodie friends, and they didn't disappoint. One of them dubbed the diet "sticks and stones" after seeing burdock—a long, thin, brown root with a wood-like appearance. The macrobiotic recipes include unfamiliar vegetables—like burdock—that are known for their health benefits. Eating out with friends and travelling also became more complicated.

Work

Staying on the diet at work went well. I brought lunch and snacks and made easy-to-eat vegetable sushi for lunch meetings.

A few people expressed interest in what I was doing, but otherwise people seemed not to notice. The following January, however, concerned that we were making free candy too accessible, I made the mistake of suggesting to the department administrator that we promote a healthy start to the year and end the practice of putting out a bowl of candy after lunch. I hadn't realized my voice carried to the nearby cubicles until they all emptied. People did not agree with my suggestion—one person complained I was trying to tell him what to eat. That wasn't my intent, but I got the message.

IMMERSION

I was curious about the rationale behind the diet and its roots in traditional Chinese medicine. When I had the time and opportunity, I took classes in topics such as the five elements theory, macrobiotic diagnosis, and the concept of yin and yang. I enjoyed the classes and found them helpful when making food choices.[5]

Diet and health consultations with the class instructors made it easier to put what I learned into practice. When their recommendations involved more cooking, I was fortunate to have help from experienced cooks.

A BROADER VIEW

In classes and elsewhere, I met a diverse community of people who were interested in health and other aspects of eating a plant-based diet. Some practiced a macrobiotic diet but made somewhat different food choices than I did depending on their preferences, constitutions, and health needs. There were also those who went back to eating meat, chicken, and dairy but continued to eat organic grains, beans, and vegetables and to limit the amount of sugar and highly processed food they ate.

Likewise, some people relied solely on macrobiotics for their

5 See the Bibliography for books by Michio Kushi and others.

health care, while others, like me, continued to see a doctor for checkups or when otherwise necessary. The checkups gave me important feedback. After I had been on the diet for several years, I learned I needed a vitamin B12 supplement.[6] I was pleased that I no longer needed to seek medication for allergies, skin rashes, and digestive problems.

GOING FORWARD

At the end of the first year, I was happy with the choice I had made. I liked the food, was comfortable with cooking, and enjoyed shopping in natural foods stores and at farmers markets. I looked forward to continuing on and was happily rewarded.

Two years later I had lost 40 pounds and was back to my high school weight of 125 pounds. After years of gaining weight, I was careful not to lose too much—my weight has now remained approximately the same for over twenty years. My skin had improved, I had more stamina, and I rarely had allergy symptoms.

THE PRESENT

The world has changed tremendously in its recognition of the effects of diet on health. There's more knowledge of how diet can affect allergies and other health problems, a growing inter-

6 Tests for my methylmalonic acid and homocysteine levels showed I needed supplemental vitamin B12.

est in plant-based diets, and access to a vast quantity of information on the Internet. YouTube videos with descriptions of plant-based food and how to cook it and online cooking classes make it easier to follow a plant-based diet. Research into the human microbiome is influencing how people view their diet and may lead to more interest in the high-fiber food that's an integral part of plant-based diets.

PLANT-BASED DIETS TODAY

With today's increased awareness of the interaction between diet and health, diet is more likely to be used to address health problems, including allergies. This has led to specialized diets becoming more popular, and a variety of plant-based diets now exist. Each has a somewhat different emphasis. Some are similar to macrobiotics, while others may be significantly different, although their roots may be in macrobiotics.

It's easier to find plant-based food now, whether you're shopping for it or dining out. Due to the growing demand for plant-based food, grocery stores and restaurants specialize in it, and plant-based options are more widely available elsewhere.

Macrobiotics has also made changes over the years. There's now more emphasis on lighter and more complex dishes that use a greater variety of plant-based ingredients than when I began the diet. For example, I now eat less brown rice and more yams or sweet potatoes, avocadoes, brown rice pasta, quinoa, and vegetable salads.

Depending on your health needs, medical and health professionals might recommend adding plant-based food to your diet instead of completely overhauling it as I did. I may not have had as much success if I had adopted a gradual approach because I had to both eliminate and add food. I benefitted from having a well-defined plan.

WHAT I DO NOW

I've followed a plant-based plus fish diet and have remained free of allergy symptoms for over twenty years. When fall comes to New England, I now look forward to the beautiful fall colors. I no longer struggle with hay fever, and I no longer have allergy symptoms in the spring. It's only when I eat too much of certain foods that I develop temporary allergic reactions, such as itchy skin.

After an uncertain beginning, I prefer plant-based food and enjoy cooking it. I'm more relaxed about my diet now. Sometimes I stay fairly close to the format of my early training in macrobiotics while at other times I eat a more varied diet of plant-based food. I buy organic food, locally grown organic vegetables and fruit when they're available, good-quality oil and sea salt, wild-caught white-meat fish and salmon, and organic rice from California. See Resources. I make healthy choices whenever possible, and I do the best I can when my options are limited. Occasionally, I explore other plant-based approaches to nutrition and experiment with the foods and techniques.

I've continued to follow the lifestyle practices described earlier in this chapter: I eat at regular mealtimes, sit down to eat, chew well, wait two to three hours after dinner before going to bed, and walk outside daily for at least thirty minutes.

In writing about my experience with allergies and diet, I've become even more aware of the impact diet has on our health and the reality that as things change, we may need to modify the diet we have become accustomed to.

CHAPTER 3
MANAGEMENT AND PROBLEM-SOLVING TECHNIQUES

If I had an hour to solve a problem
I'd spend 55 minutes thinking
about the problem and 5 minutes
thinking about solutions.

—Albert Einstein

Many of the management and problem-solving techniques used in the workplace are applicable to everyday life. Adapting those I was familiar with to transition to a new diet made it easier for me to follow the diet accurately and to stay on it over time. They helped me integrate the diet into my life not only in changing the foods I ate and in cooking more but in a broader, more realistic context that included my work schedule and lifestyle.

I had learned that for me to eliminate my allergy symptoms, it would take more than exchanging animal-based food for plant-based. I would also need to make other lifestyle changes, such as planning meals, having better eating habits, and engaging in more physical activity. I questioned whether I could find time to make these changes until I began to think of them as a system that I could control with the management and problem-solving techniques I used every day in my professional life. I realized these techniques could work just as well when applied to managing a new diet.

Over the course of your life, you have developed your own set of problem-solving techniques. In addition to the management and problem-solving tools I write about here, consider how you might apply your own experiences to tackling a new diet and entering a life-changing path.

DECISION-MAKING

Good decision-making is important to any endeavor. At home, in school, at work—we make decisions every day. Personal decisions have an emotional component that often tilts the balance in favor of the decision we like the most.

Lists of pros and cons are easy-to-use decision-making tools that allow examining decisions from more than one perspective. Pluses-and-minuses lists are a variation that lets you assign weights to the items in the list by specifying a number of pluses and minuses. At work, we used pluses-and-minuses lists when comparing alternative solutions, especially when we were faced with a difficult problem. They offered a way to clarify the problem for everyone involved as well as a way to solicit their ideas and feedback.

The pluses-and-minuses list for my diet was straightforward. Looking at the list below, the numbers of pluses and minuses are close, but since I didn't have another solution for my allergy problems, the diet had the potential to be a big plus. I also was curious to know if the diet would work for me and wanted to try it. I needed to resolve the minuses so I could manage them even if I wasn't able to turn them into pluses. Furthermore, the diet was an experiment I could stop if it didn't work out.

PLANT-BASED DIET PLUSES-AND-MINUSES LIST

++++	May alleviate allergy problems
++	May lose excess weight
++	Live a healthier lifestyle
--	Difficult to balance work schedule and meal planning and preparation
--	Social eating, entertaining, and travel more difficult
--	Give up many favorite foods

PLANNING

From my project management experience, I knew that advance planning is necessary for a project to run smoothly and to achieve its goals. I also had learned the importance of consistency in any endeavor—showing up ready to work and performing as expected. I felt the same was true for the diet and lifestyle changes I wanted to make. Although I didn't have to excel at plant-based cooking to change my diet, to succeed I would have to cook most days and do it well enough that I enjoyed cooking and eating the food I prepared.

To get started, I knew I'd need to buy different kinds of food, learn new recipes, and bring lunch to work instead of buying it in the cafeteria. I created weekly menu plans, which I used to ensure variety and for food shopping. But that was only part of the planning process. I also had to incorporate the diet into my life. Because of the classes, I was already successfully cooking plant-based food. More difficult in some ways were the situational aspects of the diet and lifestyle changes, such as finding time to walk outside every day and arranging to eat in places where I could make healthy—or at least relatively healthy—food choices when dining out or travelling.

Staying true to the diet required me to be more mindful of the end of my work day. In order to be home to cook, I made an effort to leave work on time. If I had unfinished work at the end of the day, I worked at home after dinner. When staying at work late was necessary, I arranged to eat dinner out. Occasionally, unexpected problems required me to be at work early or to stay later than planned, and I made sure to always have the ingredients available to prepare quick and easy meals. Simple things can make a big difference—bringing lunch to work was important, so I had an extra thermos jar and containers to use if I left my lunch bag at work.

My work experience also taught me the importance of backup and contingency planning. Plans don't always work out, whether in our personal lives or in a corporation. At work, we built backup and contingency plans into our normal planning. When I applied these concepts to my diet, I was better prepared for last-minute changes to my schedule. They were especially helpful at times when my life got more complicated or when travelling. Plant-based food was harder to find when eating out then, and for long trips I stayed somewhere where I could cook. Today, before leaving on a trip I use the Internet to become familiar with the area where I'll be staying. I look for local plant-based-friendly and fish restaurants and markets where I can buy food.

USING CRITICAL SUCCESS FACTORS FOR PLANNING AND PROJECT MANAGEMENT

The Critical Success Factors management technique originated to help businesses plan and manage projects, but it has benefits elsewhere. As defined by John Rockart, a professor at MIT's Sloan School of Management, who helped to popularize them, "Critical success factors are the few key areas of activity in which favorable results are absolutely necessary for a particular manager to reach his [or her] goals."

In any plan, the list of crucial elements that can make or break the plan is often very short. Using Critical Success Factors (CSFs) helps define that list. CSFs add a valuable dimension to priorities because they communicate to everyone involved in a project which tasks require special attention, and which ones aren't well-defined and need to be worked on early in the project.

When I started using Critical Success Factors at work, I discovered that my projects were more likely to be completed on schedule, including those that spanned multiple years and involved a large number of people. For all projects, I began by defining the requirements for the project to succeed and then planned accordingly, making sure that everyone involved understood the criteria for success. If we encountered problems and had to change the scope of a project, using CSFs allowed us to make better decisions about which tasks to defer or, in some cases, eliminate entirely.

During the lecture at which I first learned about Critical Success Factors, the speaker told of being asked by a client if he ever used them in his own life. He said yes, that in thinking of his own situation, he had realized he needed to spend more time with his family so he reduced the consulting work that required him to travel. Previously, he hadn't stopped to consider that even though his family was the most important thing in his life, because of his busy travel schedule, he was spending the least amount of time with them.

In my personal life, using Critical Success Factors helps with decision-making and also influences how I approach projects such as changing my diet. For instance, the Critical Success Factors I defined for my new diet were:

- To follow it accurately.
- To integrate the needs of the diet into other priorities, such as my work schedule.
- To make time to shop for food and cook.
- To walk outside daily.
- To implement the diet and lifestyle changes in a way that made following them practical and enjoyable.

As I had anticipated, my old eating habits took over from time to time, but remembering my CSFs helped me to side-step them and make healthier choices about what to eat. At times, however, I had to use other methods to deal with food cravings. When my company moved to a new building, on the way to my office in the morning I had to pass by the cafeteria at the time they were baking blueberry muffins. I couldn't resist the smell and most days bought one, no matter what I had eaten for breakfast. I had given up my old habit of buying a coffee and croissant on the way to work, but now I was developing a blueberry muffin habit. Food cravings were winning over CSFs.

I knew I had to do something about it. Muffins were not helping my allergies and finding a way to control my craving for them had become a CSF. After considering the alternatives, I made a pact with a friend who had a similar muffin problem. We vowed to give up eating all baked-flour products for three months and exchanged email every day to track our progress. The pact worked to break our muffin habits, and it also reduced our dependency on eating other baked-flour products. I discovered that what I couldn't do for myself I *could* do for my friend or to keep our pact or perhaps both. The experience taught me a lot about reducing food cravings. After several weeks, I could walk by the cafeteria in the morning without craving a blueberry muffin. Since then, with the help of CSFs, I find it easier to avoid eating food that I know isn't good for me.

PROBLEM-SOLVING

I had found it ironic that I seemed to be taking better care of my computer systems at work than of my own health. This may have been because I knew more about them. In the absence of changes in external conditions, computer systems are deterministic. They give the same response, correct or incorrect, to a specific input. We humans, however, are more complicated.

At work, I had received valuable training in solving problems from more experienced colleagues. Following their lead, I always attempted to address a problem at the time it occurred to prevent it from leading to a cascade of other problems and because if it caused a system failure, I knew the system would likely fail again—often very quickly. It was crucial to validate the suspected cause of a problem not only to prevent its recurrence, but 1) to make sure I was solving the right problem, and 2) to avoid having myths spring up about how the computer

Don't look where you fell, but where you slipped

—African Proverb

hardware and software worked. Within the limits of the available technology, my colleagues and I devised ways to deal with system vulnerabilities and limitations, and when we couldn't address a problem directly, we developed a workaround.

It wasn't necessary for me to know everything about a computer system in order to work with it successfully. When I needed to know more, I could run tests designed to give me the information, consult manuals and technical support teams, or look to colleagues for help.

I used this experience to help me manage my diet and allergies. I didn't have medical knowledge, but I did have a lifetime of personal experience and had learned enough to know what changes to look for with my diet. When I had a question, I could experiment by adjusting what I ate, refer to books, or consult with people who had more experience.

Today, I believe in prevention when possible, try to address problems when they occur, rely on the care of medical and health professionals, and look for a workaround when I'm not able to tackle a problem directly. Changing my diet and making lifestyle changes proved to be a workaround for controlling my allergies.

SYSTEMS AND SYSTEMS THINKING

The word "system" has become a catch-all for any complex structure. The Merriam-Webster dictionary defines system as: "a regularly interacting or interdependent group of items forming a unified whole." I found it helpful to view my diet as a system comprised of not only the food—although food is a major component of it—but other components, which include the lifestyle changes I've described, education, experience, and planning.

A management technique now gaining in popularity is Systems Thinking, which provides a way to understand the dynamics of complex situations and to manage them. Systems Thinking is being taught in universities as well as being applied to business, education, and elsewhere as an effective approach to problems that may not be fully defined or for which the obvious solution can result in unintended consequences. For example, when fixing a bug or adding a new feature to one component of a computer system, by understanding *all* the implications of the change, problems can be avoided in other components that on the surface seem unrelated but will be affected by the change. After more than twenty years, following my diet has become routine, yet I'm still always aware of the impact of my schedule on meals and adjust both my schedule and meal plans accordingly.

SYSTEM MONITORING

Monitoring computer systems prevents problems by providing valuable information about the demands being placed on them and is essential to keeping them running well. I've observed that computer systems are more apt to experience problems when pushed to their limits. The same holds true for people. Both people and computer systems tend to function better with reserve capacity.

Mindfulness is the process of
actively noticing new things.

—Ellen Langer

One of the first things I did when I began work each day was to look at graphs of the previous day's system usage and performance. I was looking for unusual patterns. With experience, I could differentiate between a potential problem and normal fluctuations.

Similarly, I try to observe new trends and patterns with my health. For example, I learned the rudiments of visual diagnosis, and now most mornings I quickly assess how my skin, eyes, and tongue look. With such a small amount of data, I don't bother to record what I notice, but I use the information to adjust my diet or remind myself I need more sleep, for example.

Computers start with a blank slate, and software or specialized hardware makes them functional. As the systems became larger and more complicated, my colleagues and I developed more sophisticated tools to monitor them.

We humans are equipped with systems that help us achieve homeostasis or internal stability. Most of the time, we receive warnings, such as inflammation or a fever, when something is wrong. By monitoring how we feel, how we look, and what our energy level is, often we can make adjustments to prevent problems from occurring or limit them from getting worse. Changing our diet is one such adjustment, and it can have a huge positive influence on our health.

CHAPTER 4
STAYING HEALTHY BEYOND DIET

The number of things that appear
to make people ill is exceeded only
by the number of those that claim
to make them well.

—James Harvey Robinson, "The Philosopher's
Stone," *The Atlantic Monthly*, April 1919

James Harvey Robinson's article was a tribute to F.M. Alexander and the Alexander Technique. The humorous observation he made 100 years ago easily could be made today. There might be more agreement on how to achieve good health now than there was then, but, still, there are countless opinions and everyone has their favorites. As I've described in the preceding chapters, diet and the associated lifestyle practices are my highest priority for good health. In this chapter, I discuss other health practices I rely on.

THE ALEXANDER TECHNIQUE

The Alexander Technique offers an effective way to eliminate habits that lead to unnecessary muscular tension and harmful patterns of movement. It has helped people of all ages to become better coordinated and to recover from injuries. The technique, which is taught in private lessons by teachers who have completed an approved training program,[1] is not a series of exercises or physical therapy but instead can be characterized as an educational technique that teaches people to move with more awareness and poise. It receives high praise from actors, musicians, and other performers for whom freedom of movement and mind-body awareness are so important.

I was introduced to the technique in a class that demonstrated several mind-body techniques. I quickly saw how the Alexander Technique might help me counteract the postural effects of sitting for many hours a day at my desk or in front of a computer. I began taking lessons that taught me how to avoid slumping, which not only improved my posture but also improved my breathing and contributed to a feeling of overall well-being. I found the lessons so beneficial that I completed the teacher training and continue to participate in teacher's classes.

Frederick Matthias Alexander, for whom the technique is named, was a Shakespearean actor from Australia, whose acting career was in jeopardy when he became hoarse while reciting

---

1 For further information about F. M. Alexander and the Alexander Technique, see Resources and the Bibliography.

on stage. When doctors couldn't find the cause, Alexander began a long, painstaking process of self-observation, often aided by mirrors, to figure out what he was doing differently during a performance than in everyday conversation. Alexander solved his problem in three steps: first, he saw that when he began to recite he interfered with his breathing by pulling his head back and tightening his jaw; he then discovered that being aware of this tendency wasn't enough to prevent it because he was responding habitually to the stimulus of reciting and using excess muscular tension; finally, he devised a way to stop the harmful habit by thinking preventative "directions." Following his success, his doctors in Australia dubbed him "the breathing man" and sent voice patients to him. In 1904, Alexander moved to London, where he introduced the technique to a wider audience that included many prominent people, physicians among them. Word spread, and people who had injuries and other health problems also began seeking him out to learn his technique. While in London, Alexander began a teacher training program. Today, Alexander Technique training programs can be found in many parts of the world.

> People do not decide their futures,
> they decide their habits and their
> habits decide their futures.
>
> —F. M. Alexander

MOVEMENT, CONDITIONING, AND STRENGTHENING

Movement seems to be the one thing that everyone agrees promotes better health. Whether performing micro-movements while seated, household chores such as cleaning, or more structured or intense activities, anything that gets us moving can be beneficial.

Walking—something I do every day—is easily adapted to one's fitness level. It helps with conditioning and offers many other health benefits. I also participate in other fitness activities. I took Pilates lessons for a mind-body workout and the opportunity to learn more about fitness in general. When I began strength training, my goal was to become stronger without getting hurt. I accomplished this with the help of a trainer and by approaching it with the Alexander Technique in mind.

There are many choices for adding movement to your life. You can move more in your daily routines, go to a class, join a gym, create your own home workout routine by using an online video, or all of the above. The important thing is to develop fitness goals and then shape your activities to achieve them.

INJURIES AND INFLAMMATION

Despite your best efforts, your head, feet, and everything in between can become hurt or injured. I have favorite home remedies for both, and when I don't have a remedy that works, I rely on professional health care.

My diet is to a large extent anti-inflammatory. But when I get hurt or am dealing with an injury, I'm more careful to avoid foods that contribute to inflammation and swelling. These include foods that contain sugar, baked-flour products, and other refined carbohydrates.

For severe pain or serious injuries, I seek immediate help from a professional. For less severe problems, I may first try home remedies that I've found useful. For a bruise, I might try a combination of the homeopathic remedy Arnica and ice or a tofu plaster. Tofu removes heat and is gentler than ice. It can be used on both larger areas, such as knees, and smaller areas, such as a toe, for which ice may be too strong. The simplest way to use it is to remove the water from a slice of firm tofu, wrap it in cheesecloth, and apply it directly to the injured area, covered by a towel for up to two hours or longer, changing it when it gets hot.[2]

CHIROPRACTIC CARE

More than twenty years ago, I was fortunate to learn of a chiropractor who practices "low-force" chiropractic, which works well for me. Since then, I've relied on her to help me through a variety of structural injuries. These included injuries that were relatively minor but didn't resolve on their own and those that were more serious.

2 For information about using a tofu plaster as a home remedy refer to *The Macrobiotic Path to Total Health*.

OTHER HELPFUL PRACTICES

In working with the Alexander Technique, I've seen its benefits for helping to avoid or heal injuries and other health problems. Likewise, strength training, when done properly, can help. Other practices I find helpful are yoga, shiatsu massage, and acupuncture. Occasionally, I explore other helpful health practices or wellness activities.

INDOOR POLLUTION

There are many sources of indoor pollution that can affect health and contribute to allergies; some are easier to remediate than others. I routinely open windows and use house plants and an air cleaner to help clean the air. I use natural cleaning products, avoid artificial scents, buy mattresses that are made without flame retardant chemicals, and when possible choose upholstery that is made without those chemicals.

CHAPTER 5
STORIES

I often hear stories from people who improved their health by changing their diets or who didn't have a serious health problem but feel better eating a plant-based diet. The stories below are real-world examples of how changing one's diet and lifestyle can make a big difference.

THE DISAPPEARING GALL BLADDER PROBLEM

In *Staying Healthy with the Seasons,* Dr. Elson Haas writes about traditional Chinese medicine (TCM) and how seasonal changes influence our health. TCM views the liver and gall bladder as paired organs that are more active in the spring.

It was March, springtime in New England. I had just finished reading Haas's book and felt compelled to say something when I saw a colleague, who was scheduled to have gall bladder surgery, leaving the cafeteria with an oil-laden tuna salad sandwich. When I suggested she eat something without oil that would put less stress on her gall bladder, she replied: "What should I eat?" She didn't feel well, and I knew that any recommendation I made had to be very easy to prepare and have a more relaxing effect on her liver and gall bladder than her typical diet. She listened when I suggested she stay home for a couple of days and prepare very simple meals of white rice with frozen peas and carrots. I also recommended she drink only water or non-caffeinated tea. No alcohol or sweets. The results surprised us both. Her gall bladder symptoms disappeared, and her doctor cancelled the surgery.

SUCCESS WITH A GLUTEN-FREE, PLANT-BASED DIET

Dan credits a chance meeting and the Internet with helping him transform his life with a gluten-free, plant-based diet.

A runner and reasonably healthy in high school, Dan started gaining weight after he left school and developed skin problems. By the time he reached thirty, he was overweight with bad skin and severe stomach problems that required surgery. That all changed after a chance meeting with a woman who described how she had dramatically improved her health by eliminating all gluten from her diet. As she enumerated the problems she'd resolved by changing her diet, Dan realized she could be describing him. She explained how an elimination diet could help him figure out which foods agreed with him and which didn't. Using the Internet, he learned more about elimination diets and gluten. Following this, Dan completely changed his diet and was absolutely rigorous about what he ate. He began running again, became stronger, and returned to his high school weight. He found that his skin cleared, and his stomach problems disappeared.

Dan's story is unusual for his complete commitment to his diet. He never eats food he knows is harmful for him. He's also a creative cook and uses the Internet for ideas to keep his diet interesting, often varying ingredients and cooking styles. When I asked how he manages to be so consistent with his diet, he cited two factors. First, the results are compelling; second, he tends to be independent. Dan works near home and has a flexible schedule, so he finds it relatively easy to stay on the diet during the week. Initially, weekends were a problem because his social life often involved food he no longer ate, such as pizza and beer. Over time, though, his friends made accommodations when they were together.

RESOLVING INDIGESTION AND STOMACH ACHES

Erin had always been prone to indigestion and stomach aches, which she "lived with." In college, she learned about nutrition from a roommate who was majoring in food science. Later, when Erin took a job in a busy restaurant, she changed her diet to one she had learned would give her the sustained energy she needed to get through a busy shift. To her surprise, the new diet, which included mostly plant-based food and no refined sugar or highly processed food, also relieved her digestive problems.

A CHANGE FOR THE BETTER

Tom worked seven miles from his home and commuted to work by car. When his car broke down, he began commuting by bus and on foot. Aided by a transportation app that helped him choose between two bus routes, he found he preferred his new commute and liked getting more exercise.

Despite the short driving distance from his home to work, it could take up to an hour longer than expected because of heavy traffic. Using public transportation and walking added minutes to the expected length of his commute, but was less stressful, provided exercise, and was more predictable. He continued his new routine even after his car was fixed.

Tom's story is an example of adapting to change—driving to work was becoming increasingly difficult while public transportation had improved.

WEIGHT LOSS

Lana, a private duty caregiver, wanted to know how I managed to keep my weight down. She said she was slender when she was young, but now in her 50s, she was overweight. I told her about Denny Waxman's book, *The Complete Macrobiotic Diet*.

When I saw her a few months later, she said she had read the book several times, cover to cover. She declared herself to be on a plant-based diet and was thrilled with the improvements to her skin. I was impressed by how she had translated the information in the book to a way of eating that was familiar to her from growing up eating plant-based food. She hadn't lost weight, however.

Fast-forward two years and Lana was noticeably slimmer. She told me she was walking more and said it had taken two years to achieve a noticeable weight loss. She found, though, that she was returning to eating chips, milk shakes, and other snacks, and she wished she could be more consistent with her diet. We talked about how she could add variety to her diet to make it more interesting and about healthy snacks she could bring to work.

Lana is happy with the progress she's making. She has lost weight and is on track to meeting her target weight. By paying attention to her diet and making an effort to walk every day, Lana is enjoying having more energy for work and life with her family and friends.

CONCLUSION

We make decisions about our lives every day—big and small, life-changing and not—yet we tend to hand decisions about our health over to others. That's what I frequently did until I learned how to take control of my allergies and health with diet and lifestyle changes. Relying solely on expert care from medical professionals can be life-saving when dealing with an acute medical problem. I find, however, that it's often not the best way to deal with non-acute or chronic problems; for these I find that a successful outcome depends on my active participation.

In these situations, I've learned to be mindful of how I feel and, when necessary, to adjust my diet and activity. I discovered the benefits of eating well and the damage done by eating the wrong foods and having harmful lifestyle habits. Adopting

> Life can only be understood backwards; but it must be lived forwards.
>
> —Søren Kierkegaard

a plant-based diet was the key to alleviating my allergies without medication and enjoying better overall health. In this book, I have described the dietary and lifestyle adjustments that changed my life. I have also described management techniques I used to make the transition easier. Whether you use these or adapt your own management strategies, they can—like the structural support of a building—provide a framework for successfully making dietary and other changes.

At different times in my life, circumstances put me on a path that wasn't in the mainstream. I learned to live with allergies when they were less prevalent than they are today and when their symptoms were less likely to be recognized as allergies. I began working with computers when few people knew what they were. When I was introduced to a plant-based diet as a way to control my allergy symptoms, I was comfortable with taking a new and unusual approach to solve the problem. Because for me conventional allergy remedies were only somewhat successful, I embraced an unconventional approach that promised better overall health in return for putting more time and effort into how and what I ate.

Today, plant-based diets are more common, and following one is easier. One reason for this is that there is more awareness now of the major impact diet has on health—and especially on allergies. In response, a greater variety of plant-based foods is available in grocery stores and restaurants. Scientific advances in related areas, such as the microbiome and gut bacteria, offer promises for further understanding in the future.

At one time, I would have said cooking at home is essential

for eating a healthy plant-based diet. Today, however, although I still believe it makes a difference, whether or not it's necessary may depend on a person's health and the resources that are available to them. I've met people who seem to manage the diet while eating most of their meals out and buying prepared food. Still, to successfully follow a plant-based or primarily plant-based diet for many years requires maintaining a dietary balance that makes cooking at home beneficial.

When I couldn't resolve a computer problem by direct means, such as when I bumped up against the limits of technology, I looked for a good workaround. Changing my diet was a good workaround for eliminating my allergy problems, and it is one that has had many other benefits. Over the years, I've observed that:

- Learning about diet and health is a lifelong investment that pays big dividends.
- Good health begins with food selection and the choices we make.
- When making dietary changes, it's important to be mindful of maintaining a healthy balance of food that provides the stamina needed each day. Simply eliminating parts of a meal, such as avoiding orange juice at breakfast because of its sugar content, can lead to feeling hungry and being susceptible to snacking. Instead, finding a substitute is healthier and more satisfying. For example, in the case of breakfast adding leafy greens or choosing a different menu is a better way to start the day.

- Chewing is an important part of eating. I recently noticed someone chewing very well who said he wasn't aware of it but that his parents often complained about how slowly he ate. His health was better for it, and he was fortunate that he hadn't changed what was a naturally healthy habit.
- In general, but especially when making dietary and other lifestyle changes, it helps to take a bit of time every day to note the direction of your health—is it better, worse, or the same as yesterday—and to pay attention to what works well and what doesn't.

Making the decision to be healthier is one of the best things you can do for yourself. Changing your diet can change the way you feel, and feeling good every day is revitalizing. My great-aunt Sadie would have agreed. I hope this book inspires you to discover a healthier, happier you!

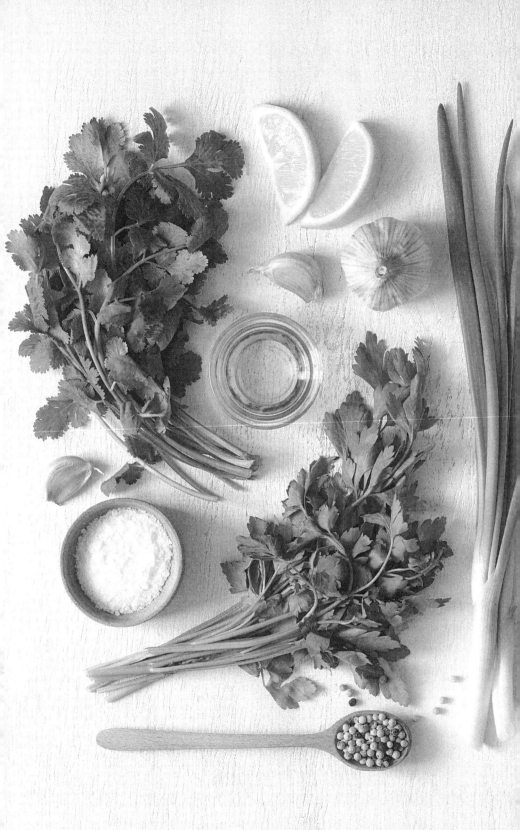

PART 2

COOKING, MENUS, AND RECIPES

CHAPTER 6
LIGHTLY COOKED LEAFY GREEN VEGETABLES

I was familiar with lettuce and other salad greens when I began a plant-based diet, but not with the denser, dark leafy greens such as collard greens and kale. These greens are delicious as a separate or side dish, not only as an ingredient in other dishes such as soup or a stir fry. Simple dishes of leafy greens are easy to prepare and when they're lightly cooked the greens have a lovely bright color and fresh taste. I find them a welcome addition to meals.

Nutritionally, leafy greens are high in fiber, vitamins, and minerals. Lightly cooking them makes them more digestible while preserving their nutritional value. I cook leafy greens most days, often eating them for breakfast. I choose from a variety of greens that include curly kale, lacinato (dinosaur) kale, bok choy, collard greens, mustard greens, napa cabbage, and watercress.

PREPARATION

After washing the greens thoroughly, use a knife to remove bad spots and trim the stems as needed. I use a vegetable knife and a wooden or bamboo cutting board. For further information about vegetable knives and cutting boards see Chapter 2, Next Steps to a New Diet: Setting Up a Plant-Based Kitchen.

Bok Choy: Cut the white stem and leaves into bite-size pieces and place them in separate bowls. When cooking, add the stem to the water a bit before the leaves.

Collard Greens: Lay the leaf flat and cut the stem away from the center. The leaves can be stacked and cut into bite-size rectangles or rolled and cut into thin strips. Cut the pieces into similar sizes so they'll cook evenly. The stem is nutritious and can be used by finely chopping it and cooking it with the leaves. Add the stem to the water a minute or so before the leaves, depending on its thickness.

You can make green vegetable rolls with collard greens by first cooking several whole leaves with the stem cut out, then draining them and laying the cooked leaves flat, overlapping them. Add cooked, sliced mushrooms, matchstick cut carrots, or other filling. Roll like sushi and slice. The cooking time for the leaves depends on their size and thickness. You can tell when they're ready by their color and texture.

Curly Kale and Lacinato (Dinosaur) Kale: Cut like collard greens or, using your hands, hold the stem with one hand and remove the leaves into a bowl with the other. Tear the leaves into bite-sized pieces. As with collards, you can finely chop the stem and cook with the leaves.

Mustard Greens: See Kale. Mustard greens have a naturally bitter, pungent flavor.

Napa Cabbage: See Bok Choy

Watercress: Watercress is an aquatic plant and may require careful washing before cooking. Like mustard greens, it has a naturally bitter flavor.

Other Greens: You can use the stems and leafy tops of daikon radish and turnip greens. After washing them well, finely chop, and steam, adding the stems to the water before the leaves. The cooking time will vary depending on their thickness. With so many other choices available, I don't often eat spinach and chard. While they have nutritional benefits, they also contain oxalate, which interferes with calcium absorption.[1]

COOKING

To keep meals interesting, I vary the types of greens and cooking styles. With a little practice, you'll learn to adjust cooking times to their thickness and freshness. You'll also discover that

1 Harvard Health Newsletter, June 2009

the taste of the greens varies depending on their freshness and that the greens can become bitter when overcooked.

QUICK BOILING

Bring the water to boiling and add a few grains of sea salt. Cooking with too much salt makes the greens bitter.

Quick-boil the greens until they turn a bright green, usually about 30 to 60 seconds or longer, depending on their thickness and freshness. I use a long-handled mesh strainer to remove them from the pot.

When quick-boiling, I often use more than one vegetable and type of vegetable—leafy green, round, and root—to make a boiled salad. Cook the vegetables one at a time in the same pot of water starting with the mildest vegetable first. Bring the water back to boiling between vegetables.

STEAMING

Steam only one vegetable at a time for one to three minutes depending on its thickness and freshness. Salt isn't necessary when steaming. Steamed greens should retain some of their crunchiness and be a bright but somewhat darker color than when boiled. Any steamer will work, but I like to use a steamer pot that's similar to a double-boiler.

OTHER COOKING METHODS

In addition to quick-boiling and steaming, I oil sauté, water sauté, or sauté with a combination of oil and water.

DRESSINGS

I sometimes use a squeeze of lemon, a dash of vinegar, or a salad dressing. A simply prepared dish of leafy greens balances more complex dishes in a meal.

LEFTOVERS

Because leafy greens are best when they're freshly cooked, I cook only the amount I plan to use.

SHOPPING FOR LEAFY GREENS

When shopping for leafy greens, I select the freshest organic greens I can find. Freshness and quality affect their taste and nutrition.

CHAPTER 7
SAMPLE MENU PLAN AND RECIPES

Growing up I loved to eat but wasn't interested in cooking. After leaving home, out of necessity I cooked staples from the meals I had watched my mother prepare. These included egg omelets; meat, chicken, and fish dishes; potatoes, pasta, and salad; and canned, frozen, or fresh vegetables depending on the season. Occasionally, I tried cooking food from French or other cuisines and baking. My go-to desserts were apple pie, chocolate chip cookies, and frosted mint-chocolate brownies, one of my mother's favorite recipes that everyone loved.

All that changed, however, after I learned to cook plant-based food and became more interested in cooking. Today, I enjoy cooking, use healthy, colorful ingredients, and cook nearly every day. Desserts are likely to be stewed fruit or puddings sweetened with apple juice, and I occasionally bake almond cookies or apple crisps made without refined sugar. My main sources for recipes are classes, cookbooks, and online resources. Most days, I cook a variety of dishes, simply prepared, and cook more elaborate dishes on weekends or for special occasions.

MENU PLANNING

Menu planning, which at first seemed like a lot of work, soon became easier and enjoyable as I experimented with recipes and planned my weekly menus around healthy meals. At some point, I realized I no longer needed a detailed plan for every meal, but having even a casual plan for the week helps me to ensure that I'm eating a variety of food.

As described in Chapter 2, my guidelines for menu-planning are:

- Plan meals around whole grains and grain products along with a variety of vegetables, beans, fruit, and other plant-based food
- Vary ingredients and cooking styles
- Avoid refined sugar and limit other natural sweeteners
- Avoid highly processed food
- Be mindful of the season and weather

SAMPLE MENU PLAN OVERVIEW

The menu plan featured on pages 94–95 is for four days in late fall. It has heartier and more warming dishes than it would during the summer when I prepare a larger selection of lighter food, such as vegetable salads or grain-and-vegetable salads. On the coldest days, I'm more likely to prepare a heartier porridge in the morning and long-cooked, baked, and roasted dishes for lunch and dinner.

Today, smoothies and protein drinks are popular with people eating a variety of different diets. I haven't included them in my diet because, although they can contain a lot of nutrients and be very tasty, chewing vegetables and fruit generally is better for digestion. Depending on the ingredients, smoothies can be high in sugar that is quickly absorbed into the bloodstream and can adversely affect one's blood sugar balance.

Breakfast

On most weekdays, I follow the format described in Chapter 2, Next Steps to a New Diet: Menu Planning. On weekends, I may cook food that takes more time to prepare, such as scrambled tofu. (See recipe on page 129.) Breakfast can include:

- Grain porridge, sometimes with cooked beans added (I choose from among several grains, such as brown rice, millet, barley, and oats[1], or cook rice porridge by adding water to pre-cooked brown rice.)

---

1 People with allergies or food sensitivities may, at times, find oats to be mucus-forming.

- Quinoa
- A condiment, such as gomashio or shiso powder
- A steamed sourdough bread sandwich (See recipe on page 131.)
- Cooked vegetables, often leafy greens
- Pickles

People interested in my diet often ask what I eat for breakfast. As I describe my typical breakfast, the blank stares I get make me feel as if I'm speaking a foreign language. People find eating leafy green vegetables and grain porridges other than oatmeal for breakfast unimaginable. They're surprised to learn that at one time grain porridge was a breakfast staple across the United States. If you research breakfast by country online you'll find an interesting variety of food choices represented.

Lunch

On most weekdays I eat leftovers from the previous day's dinner following the format described in Chapter 2, Next Steps to a New Diet: Menu Planning. Lunch can include:

- A grain or noodle dish
- A vegetable dish
- Soup or a bean dish
- Pickles (some days)
- Dessert (some days)

Dinner

Dinner follows the format described in Chapter 2, Next Steps to a New Diet: Menu Planning. Dinner includes:

- Soup
- A grain or a noodle dish
- A short-cooked vegetable dish (typically under 5 minutes)
- A long-cooked vegetable dish (typically 20 minutes or longer)
- A bean dish (unless I'm making a bean soup), a dish made with a soy product such as tempeh, or fish
- Pickles or sauerkraut (some days)
- Dessert (some days)

Snacks

For snacks, I generally eat nuts, seeds, raw or cooked fruit[2], and raw or cooked sweet vegetables to which I sometimes add hummus or guacamole.

SHOPPING

I go grocery shopping weekly and often shop more than once a week for fresh vegetables and other fresh food. My shopping list is based on the weekly menu plan. I modify the plan, however, depending on which vegetables and fruit are available and which I find the most appealing. I always keep a variety of grains and beans stocked so I easily can change the plan based on the fresh food that's available.

---

2 Lightly cooking fruits and vegetables may be helpful for people who are sensitive to oral allergy syndrome, also known as pollen-food syndrome, which is caused by cross-reacting allergens found in both pollen and raw fruits, vegetables, and some tree nuts. Oral allergy syndrome can cause symptoms such as tingling on the tongue or numb lips.

SAMPLE MENU PLAN FOR LATE FALL

DAY 1	DAY 2

Breakfast

Scrambled Tofu

Steamed Whole Wheat
Sourdough Bread

Lunch

[Eat Out]

Baked Fish

Jasmine Rice

Broccoli

Dinner

Creamy Squash Soup

Medium-Grain Brown Rice with
Toasted Almonds

Carrot, Cabbage, and Turnip
Nishime

Mixed Green Salad

Fruit Kanten

Breakfast

Millet with Squash

Shiso Condiment

Steamed Kale with Lemon

Lunch

[From Dinner Day 1]

Creamy Squash Soup

Brown Rice with Toasted
Almonds

Carrot, Cabbage, and Turnip
Nishime

Dinner

Barley Stew

Arame with Carrots
and Onions

Bok Choy—oil sauté

Radish Pickles

Fruit Kanten

SAMPLE MENU PLAN AND RECIPES

| DAY 3 | DAY 4 |

Breakfast

Millet with Squash

Shiso Condiment

Steamed Collards with Lemon

Lunch

[From Dinner Day 2]

Barley Stew

Arame with Carrots and Onions

Radish Pickles

Dinner

Miso Soup

Mixed-Grain Brown Rice

Black Bean Stew

Carrot and Burdock Kinpira

Collard Greens—oil sauté

Stewed Tree Fruit

Breakfast

Grain and Sweet Vegetable Porridge

Quick-boiled Collards

Kale and Cabbage with Umeboshi Vinegar

Lunch

[From Dinner Day 3]

Mixed-Grain Brown Rice

Black Bean Stew

Carrot and Burdock Kinpira

Stewed Tree Fruit

Dinner

Noodles with Tofu and Vegetables

Mixed Green Salad

RECIPE NOTES

These recipes correspond to the meals found in the menu plan on pages 94–95. Special kitchenware requirements are listed at the beginning of each recipe. Basic kitchenware not listed includes: saucepans and skillets, measuring cups for solid ingredients and liquids, strainers, knives, a vegetable peeler, and a stove top heat diffuser. For a description of kitchenware that is particularly helpful for preparing plant-based meals, such as a vegetable knife and a stove top heat diffuser, see Chapter 2, Next Steps to a New Diet: Setting Up a Plant-Based Kitchen.

All plant-based diets emphasize vegetables, grains, beans, fruit, nuts, and seeds. They include little or no animal products. The differences between macrobiotic, vegan, and vegetarian diets are:

Macrobiotic Diet

- Plant-based with occasional fish.
- No refined sugar or highly processed food.
- Sea salt is used in cooking and salt is not added after cooking. You might see a condiment such as gomashio, which is made by grinding roasted sesame seeds and sea salt, on the dining table, but you won't find a salt shaker.
- Eating locally-grown food or food from a similar climate is recommended.
- Regular use of sea vegetables, such as arame, dulse, and kombu (also known as kelp), is recommended.

- Vegetable dishes with a Japanese influence, such as kinpira and nishime, are included.
- Limiting baked-flour products is recommended.
- Cold or iced drinks are not recommended because they interfere with digestion.
- More lightly cooked and fewer raw vegetables and fruit are recommended. The amount of raw food varies, depending on someone's health and susceptibility to pollen allergies.
- Cooking with a gas stove is recommended.

Vegan Diet

- Plant-based with no animal food.
- Includes refined sugar and processed food.
- Note: Specific diets may include other recommendations.

Vegetarian Diet

- Plant-based with dairy products.
- Includes refined sugar and processed food.
- May include eggs.
- Note: Specific diets may include other recommendations.

RECIPES

Arame with Carrots and Onions

Arame is a small sea vegetable that's a member of the kelp family. It has a somewhat sweet taste and goes well with sweet vegetables. Arame is packed with minerals and has many health benefits. It's sold dried in shredded pieces that are re-constituted by soaking them in water. Note that arame and other sea vegetables tend to be relatively high in sodium and are typically served in small quantities. Serve warm.

Serves 3 to 4

Ingredients

Approximately ½ ounce dried arame
1½ to 2 cups onions sliced into thin half-moons
Small pinch of sea salt
1 to 1¼ cups carrots sliced into thin matchsticks
¼ to ½ teaspoon shoyu
½ teaspoon juice from grated ginger (optional)

Instructions

1. Soak the arame for a few minutes until soft, strain, and discard soaking water. After soaking, use a knife to shorten any pieces that are longer than approximately 3 inches.

2. Place the onions in a medium-size skillet or saucepan, cover with water, and cook on a medium-low flame.

3. Add salt after the onions begin to soften and cook for 3 minutes.

4. Layer the carrots and then the arame on top of the onions.

5. Add water so that it reaches to the base of the arame.

6. Cover and bring to a boil on medium-high heat.

7. Lower heat and simmer for 20 to 25 minutes. Add more liquid if necessary. There should be a little liquid left in the pan for Step 9.

8. Add the shoyu and stir gently to blend the ingredients.

9. Cover and simmer on low for 5 minutes. Remove the cover and cook until most of the liquid is gone.

10. Stir to combine the ingredients.

11. Add the ginger juice if using and stir gently.

Variations: Add lotus root that's been peeled, thinly sliced, and cut into quarter-rounds on top of the carrots in Step 4. Garnish with toasted sesame seeds.

Barley and Vegetable Stew

A light, calming, and tasty stew. Adding beans can make it the centerpiece of a meal. Serve warm.

Serves 4

Essential Cookware

- Use a 2 or 2½ quart pot.
- Cooks best in a heavy pot with a tight-fitting lid.

Ingredients

1 cup pearled barley

1-inch-square piece kombu (kelp) rinsed to remove the excess salt

¼ to ½ cup diced carrots

¼ to ½ cup finely sliced celery

1 or 2 dried shitake mushrooms that have been softened by soaking them in enough water to cover them and sliced. Reserve the soaking water to use if additional water is needed during cooking (optional)

Pinch of sea salt

¼ to ½ cup finely sliced leeks

1 cup pre-cooked navy beans with ¼ to ½ cup liquid (optional)

½ to 1 teaspoon barley miso

Preliminary Preparation

Wash the barley and soak 6 to 8 hours or overnight in 2 cups of water. Strain the barley and reserve the soaking water for cooking.

To Make the Stew

1. Place the kombu and barley in the pot followed by the carrots, celery, and mushrooms.

2. Add the reserved soaking water and cover.

3. Bring to a boil and add salt.

4. Lower heat and simmer for 30 to 45 minutes until the barley is soft. Add more water if necessary.

5. Add the leeks and beans if using. Simmer for 10 minutes or until the leeks become tender.

6. Dissolve the barley miso in a small bowl of the cooking liquid and add to the pot. Simmer without bringing to a boil for 5 minutes.

Variation: Use different sweet vegetables, such as onions, carrots, cabbage, or winter squash.

Black Bean Stew

I love bean stews, and black bean stew is one of my favorites—it's tasty and energizing. Black bean stew can be prepared with many different vegetables and seasonings. While I prefer to cook the beans, I use pre-cooked canned beans when I haven't planned ahead. Pre-soaking beans reduces their cooking time and makes them more digestible as does cooking them with kombu (kelp). Serve warm.

Serves 3 to 4

Essential Cookware

- Use a 2 or 2½ quart pot.
- Cooks best in a heavy pot with a tight-fitting lid.

Cooked Beans

1 cup dried beans that have been pre-soaked

1-inch-square piece of kombu (kelp) rinsed to remove the excess salt

Bay leaf (optional)

Preliminary Preparation

Sort beans to remove any stones or debris, wash, and soak for 6 to 8 hours or overnight covered with a sushi mat or loose-weave towel. Strain the beans, rinse, and use fresh water for cooking.

Instructions

1. Place beans in pot with kombu (kelp) and a bay leaf if using.

2. Add water to cover about an inch above the beans.

3. Cover and bring to a boil, skimming off foam as it rises to the top of the pot with a long-handled fine-mesh strainer.

4. Continue boiling and, when there is no more foam, reduce flame and place the heat diffuser under the pot.

   Tip: Alternatively, pre-heat the heat diffuser on a separate burner on low heat while the ingredients in the pot are being brought to a boil. Then gently place the pot on the diffuser.

5. Simmer covered for 45 minutes or until the beans are tender but not mushy. Add water as needed during cooking to cover the beans.

Subsituting with Canned Beans

I use Eden organic canned beans which are made with kombu. Note that a 16-ounce can of black beans makes about 2 cups with the liquid or 1½ cups without.

Making Bean Stew

Note: The ratio of beans to vegetables and seasonings in a bean stew doesn't have to be exact. The measurements for the recipe below are approximate. The recipe calls for 1½ cups of cooked beans. If you've cooked one cup of dried beans you'll have about 2½ cups of cooked beans and can use the entire amount, adjusting the vegetables and seasonings and cooking in a larger pot, or use the leftover beans in another dish.

Ingredients

½ to 1 teaspoon olive or sesame oil

½ to ¾ cup diced onion

1 teaspoon minced ginger (optional)

½ to ¾ cup diced carrots

¼ cup finely sliced celery

½ to ¾ cup peeled and diced winter squash

1½ cups black beans

½ teaspoon cumin

A pinch to ¼ teaspoon sea salt or to taste

Parsley for garnish

Instructions

1. Heat oil in a saucepan or skillet and sauté onions and ginger for several minutes. Add vegetables and sauté for 5 minutes longer adding a little liquid from the beans if necessary.

2. Add beans and seasonings and cook covered for 10 minutes until flavors have blended and vegetables are tender. Adjust liquid if necessary so the dish is moist.

3. Stir gently, adjust seasonings and garnish with parsley.

Variations: Add garlic or other seasonings, or use different vegetables such as parsnips, turnips, or lotus root. Sauté onions and ginger in water instead of oil. Add water to leftover bean stew to make a bean soup. Mashing some of the stew will make a thicker soup.

Brown Rice

Brown rice is satisfying and nutritious! Chewier than white rice, it has a somewhat nutty flavor. It's a whole grain that's minimally processed to remove only the inedible outer husk, leaving the beneficial fiber and nutritious vitamins and minerals in the outer layers. Like white rice, brown rice comes in short-grain, medium-grain, and long-grain varieties, which differ in size and density. Short-grain brown rice is smaller, rounder, and denser than the medium-grain and long-grain varieties. I cook with all varieties depending on the recipe and the qualities I'm looking for, such as heartier or lighter. I most often cook short-grain or medium-grain, sometimes mixed with another variety of brown rice or another grain. I use long-grain rice when I want a lighter, less dense brown rice, and I use white rice when I want a still lighter rice, for example to accompany a meal with fish. Serve warm or at room temperature.

Boiled Brown Rice

I often boil rice, which is a lighter method of cooking than using a pressure cooker. Note that this recipe is for stovetop cooking and not for a rice cooker.

Serves 4

Essential Cookware

- Use a 2 or 2½ quart pot.
- Cooks best in a heavy pot with a tight-fitting lid.
- A wooden rice paddle is helpful for removing the rice to a serving dish.

Ingredients

1 cup organic short-grain or medium-grain brown rice (See Resources)
Small pinch of sea salt

Washing and Soaking Brown Rice

1. Wash rice in cold water, swishing it around several times to remove dust or any small stones and other debris, then drain. Repeat twice and rinse with cold water.

2. Soak rice in 2 cups of water overnight covered with a bamboo mat or loose-weave towel.

3. Strain the rice, rinse, and use fresh water for cooking.

Cooking Brown Rice

1. Place the pre-soaked rice in the pot with 2 cups of water.

2. Cover, bring to a boil, and add salt.

3. Place the heat diffuser under the pot.

   Tip: Alternatively, pre-heat the heat diffuser on a separate burner at low heat while rice is being brought to a boil and then gently place the pot on the diffuser.

4. Simmer for 50 to 55 minutes on low heat then let stand for 5 to 10 minutes.

5. Mix rice gently and transfer to a bowl. If using a rice paddle, wet it with water to prevent the rice from sticking to it.

6. Cover with a bamboo mat or loose-weave towel to keep warm.

Variations: Brown rice is very versatile and can be prepared in many different ways. Note that slight adjustments in the amount of water may be needed, especially when mixing different varieties of brown rice or brown rice with other grains.

Mixing different varieties of brown rice: Mix two or three varieties of brown rice, such as sweet rice or long-grain varieties like jasmine or basmati.

To mix with other grains: Brown rice mixes well with millet, barley, and other grains. For example, mix ¾ cup brown rice with ¼ cup millet. Grains that require soaking can be soaked together with the brown rice. Mix other grains with the rice after it's soaked.

For fall and winter entertaining: Mix 1 cup of the long-grain varieties, such as brown basmati, with ½ cup wild rice and boil in 2½ to 2¾ cups of water for 50 minutes. When done, add toasted pecans and dried cranberries that have been simmered in the juice of an orange over low heat for 5 to 10 minutes. For a combination of 1 cup of brown rice and ½ cup of wild rice, I use approximately one-third cup each of cranberries and pecans.

To make a rice salad for summer picnics: Add vegetables, such as cooked corn kernels and chopped toasted almonds, to a long-grain variety.

Pressure-Cooked Brown Rice

As its name implies, pressure-cooking is a stronger way of cooking rice than boiling and is especially nourishing in colder weather. Note that this recipe is for a stovetop pressure cooker.

Serves 4 to 5

Essential Cookware

• A 4-liter pressure cooker works well for this recipe. Use a larger pressure cooker for a larger quantity of rice.

Ingredients

1½ cups organic short-grain or medium-grain organic rice
2¼ cups water
Small pinch of sea salt

Pressure Cooking Brown Rice

1. Follow washing and soaking instructions for boiled rice.

2. Place rice, water, and salt in the pressure cooker.

3. Cover pressure cooker and bring up to pressure over medium-high heat.

4. Place the heat diffuser under pot and lower flame or move to burner with heat diffuser as described for boiled rice.

5. Cook for 45 to 50 minutes.

6. Remove from burner and let pressure come down.

7. When pressure is down, open lid and transfer to a bowl following the instructions for boiled rice.

Creamy Squash Soup

Cream soups are tasty, relaxing, and nourishing. This plant-based version of a pureed cream of squash soup is easy to prepare and satisfying. Serve hot.

Serves 3 to 4

Essential Cookware

• Use a 2 or 2½ quart pot
• Requires an immersion blender or equivalent

Ingredients

1 to 2 teaspoons olive or sesame oil

1 to 1½ cups diced onions

½ to 1 teaspoon minced ginger (optional)

3 to 4 cups winter squash, such as kabocha, buttercup, or butternut, cut into 2-inch cubes. If using organic squash, it's not necessary to peel it; however, unpeeled kabocha squash will add a greenish tint to the soup.

Sea salt to taste

Cumin to taste (optional)

Parsley (optional)

Instructions

1. Heat oil in the pot and sauté onions and ginger with a small pinch of salt until the onions start to brown.

2. Add squash with enough water to cover it.

3. Cover pot and bring to a boil over medium-high heat, reduce flame, and simmer for 15 to 20 minutes or until the squash becomes tender.

4. Remove from heat and puree with an immersion blender until the soup is smooth and creamy. Add more water if necessary to get the desired texture. (Note: if using an appliance other than an immersion blender to puree the soup, follow the instructions for that appliance.)

5. Season with salt and cumin if using.

6. Return pot to the stove, bring to a boil on medium heat, and simmer for 10 minutes.

7. Garnish with parsley.

   Tip: When choosing a kabocha squash look for one that's relatively heavy for its size, has a small navel, and has some orange or yellow on it.

Variations: Use water to sauté the onions instead of oil. Add an apple that's been peeled, cored, and chopped to make a squash and apple soup. Vary garnishes: for example, chopped pecans or pecans and sage sautéed in a little shoyu. Pureed vegetable soups can be made from single root and round vegetables, such as parsnips, cauliflower, broccoli, and carrots, or from a combination like carrot and sweet potato. Note that leftover pureed vegetable soup can be kept refrigerated and reheated for one or two days.

Fruit Kanten

Fruit kanten is a light, refreshing dessert that can be made at any time of the year using tree fruit, citrus fruit, or seasonal fruit such as berries. Serve at room temperature or cold.

Serves 2 to 3

Ingredients

1 tablespoon agar-agar flakes
1 cup apple juice or apple juice mixed with water
Small pinch of sea salt
Approximately ½ cup of berries or other fruit

Instructions

1. Place agar-agar flakes in a saucepan with the apple juice and let sit for 15 to 20 minutes. This will help the agar-agar to dissolve more quickly during cooking.

2. Wash fruit, cutting if necessary, and place in a small-to-medium-sized bowl.

3. Add salt to the contents of the saucepan and bring to a boil over medium heat, then lower heat and simmer until the agar-agar is dissolved stirring constantly.

4. Pour liquid into bowl over fruit.

5. Refrigerate when cool to set.

Variations: Use different fruit juices or combinations of fruit. Use a combination of juice and water for a less sweet dessert.

Grain and Vegetable Porridge

Comfort food at its best, this hearty porridge is warming in cool weather. Serve hot.

Serves 3 to 4

Essential Cookware

- Use a 2 or 2½ quart pot.
- Cooks best in a heavy pot with a tight-fitting lid.

Ingredients

¼ cup short- or medium-grain brown rice (soaked overnight)

¼ cup barley (soaked overnight)

¼ cup quinoa (does not require soaking)

½ to ¾ cup parsnips

A pinch to ¼ teaspoon sea salt

½ to 1 teaspoon minced ginger (optional)

3½ cups water

Preliminary Preparation

Wash the grains and soak overnight. (For information about washing and soaking the grains, see the Brown Rice recipe.)

Cooking the Porridge

1. Peel the parsnips and cut into large pieces.

2. Place the rice, barley, quinoa, parsnips, and water in pot.

3. Cover, bring to a boil, and add salt.

4. Place the heat diffuser under the pot.

   Tip: Alternatively, pre-heat the heat diffuser on a separate burner at low heat while the ingredients in the pot are being brought to a boil. Then gently place the pot on the diffuser.

5. Cook for 45 minutes to 1 hour. The porridge should be creamy, so you may have to add water toward the end of cooking.

Variations: Use different combinations of grains or one or more sweet vegetables, such as onions, carrots, cabbage, or winter squash.

Millet with Winter Squash

As a grain with dinner or as porridge for breakfast, millet, a seed-like grain, combined with winter squash or other sweet vegetables is strengthening and satisfying. Serve warm.

Serves 2 to 3

Essential Cookware

• Use a 1½ quart pot or larger.

Ingredients

½ cup millet

1 cup winter squash, such as kabocha, buttercup, or butternut, peeled and cut into bite-size chunks. If using organic squash you can leave the skin on.

Small pinch of sea salt

Shiso powder condiment (optional)

Preliminary Preparation

Wash the millet and soak in 2 to 2¼ cups of water for 6 to 8 hours or overnight. Strain the millet and reserve the soaking water for cooking.

Instructions

1. Place the millet and squash in the pot.

2. Add soaking water and cover.

3. Bring to a boil and add salt.

4. Place the heat diffuser under the pot.

   Tip: Alternatively, pre-heat the heat diffuser on a separate burner at low heat while the ingredients in the pot are being brought to a boil and then gently place the pot on the diffuser.

5. Simmer for 30 minutes. The millet should be soft and creamy, so you may have to add water towards the end of cooking.

6. Gently blend the squash and millet with a spoon.

7. Sprinkle with shiso powder condiment and serve.

Variations: Use a different condiment or different combinations of one or more vegetables, such as cauliflower, onions, and cauliflower, or onions and winter squash.

Miso Soup

This savory soup made with miso, a fermented soybean paste, is a broth-like soup that stimulates digestion and energizes the body. Serve hot

Serves 2

Ingredients

2-inch piece of wakame sea vegetable

¼ cup finely sliced onion

1 to 1½ teaspoons organic barley miso

Finely sliced scallions for garnish

Instructions

1. Rinse the wakame and soak in a little water until soft. Discard the soaking water and dice the wakame.

2. Place wakame in a saucepan with 2¼ cups of water and bring to a boil.

3. Add onions and bring to a boil. Reduce flame and simmer for about 10 minutes or until onions are soft.

4. Reduce flame to low.

5. Dissolve miso in a little of the cooking liquid and stir it into the pot.

6. Simmer uncovered for several minutes, keeping the flame low enough that the soup doesn't boil in order to preserve the beneficial enzymes in the miso.

7. Place into bowls and garnish with scallions.

Variations: Use different types of miso (sweet or savory) or combinations of one or more vegetables, such as carrots, napa cabbage, or winter squash. At the start of cooking add a dried shitake mushroom that has been soaked in water until soft and then sliced.

Mixed Green Salad

Lettuce and other raw salad ingredients are refreshing and cooling whether on a warm summer day or at other times of the year as a light addition to a meal.

Ingredients

One or more red radishes

Umeboshi vinegar

One or more heads of different kinds of lettuce (red or green leaf, romaine, butter, or iceberg)

Olive Oil

Sea salt (optional)

Instructions

1. Wash radishes. Peel non-organic radishes. Organic radishes can be left unpeeled but with bad spots removed. Cut into thin slices and marinate in umeboshi vinegar for 10 to 15 minutes.

2. Remove the lettuce leaves you plan to use, wash, and remove excess water.

3. Tear the lettuce into bite-size pieces and place in a bowl.

4. Add a little olive oil to taste.

5. Add the radishes and umeboshi vinegar

6. For a saltier taste, add additional umeboshi vinegar or a small pinch of sea salt.

Variations: There are numerous salad variations. Use different dressings or combinations of lettuce, adding tangy or bitter lettuces, such as arugula and radicchio. Add other vegetables, such as red onion, toasted walnuts or pecans, toasted squash seeds, or crumbled tofu.

Noodles and Vegetables Stir Fry

Noodles with vegetables are popular in many cuisines whether in a soup or in dishes such as Italian pasta primavera, Asian stir-fried noodles and vegetables, or noodles and vegetables in a savory broth. These dishes are flavorful, versatile, and can be the centerpiece of a meal. They're a great way to use the vegetables you have on hand. Serve warm.

Serves 3 to 4

Ingredients

Approximately 4 ounces extra-firm tofu (optional)

½ to 1 tablespoon sesame or other oil

½ to 1 cup sliced red or yellow onions

½ to 1 cup carrots cut into fine matchsticks

½ to 1½ teaspoons minced ginger (optional)

½ to 1 cup shredded cabbage

½ to 1 cup pre-cooked steamed broccoli cut into bite-size pieces

2 to 3 cups of pre-cooked noodles of your choice (wheat pasta, gluten-free pasta, Japanese udon or soba).

Pinch of sea salt

¼ to ½ teaspoon of shoyu

¼ teaspoon umeboshi vinegar (optional)

Instructions

1. Prepare the tofu if using. (See steps 1 and 2 of the recipe for scrambled tofu).

2. In a wok or skillet, heat the oil and sauté onions, carrots, and ginger for a few minutes.

3. Crumble the tofu or cut it into cubes and add with a little more oil.

4. Stir-fry until onions are translucent.

5. Add cabbage with 2 to 3 tablespoons of water.

6. Stir-fry until cabbage is tender.

7. Add pre-cooked broccoli and noodles.

8. Season with salt, shoyu, and umeboshi vinegar and add ¼ cup water as needed.

9. Continue to stir-fry for two minutes to adjust the taste and the amount of water.

Variations: Sauté with water instead of oil. Use different combinations of vegetables and seasonings.

Radish Pickles

Pickles aid digestion and are a tasty addition to any meal whether breakfast, lunch, or dinner.

Essential Cookware

- 8- to 12-ounce glass jar, such as a mason jar
- Cheesecloth to cover jar
- String or rubber band

Ingredients

1 to 2 cups of red radishes
Umeboshi vinegar

Instructions

1. Wash radishes. Peel non-organic radishes. Organic radishes can be left unpeeled but with bad spots removed. Cut into thin slices.

2. Place radishes in the jar so they fill it to the top.

3. Mix the umeboshi vinegar with water in the ratio of 1 part vinegar to 3 parts water and add to the jar, making sure the liquid covers the radishes.

4. Cover the jar with cheesecloth and use string or a rubber band to hold it in place.

5. Leave at room temperature for 12 to 24 hours, replace the cheesecloth with the jar lid, and put in the refrigerator.

6. Rinse before eating if you want pickles that are less salty.

7. The pickles will keep refrigerated for 7 to 10 days.

Variation: Use other vegetables, thinly sliced, such as daikon radish and red top or Hakurei turnips.

Root Vegetable Sauté Kinpira Style

A dish with Japanese origins, kinpira style root vegetables are nutritious and flavorful. Serve warm.

Serves 4 to 6

Ingredients

1 teaspoon sesame oil

1 cup burdock root, gently washed with a vegetable brush, and cut into thin matchsticks

1 cup lotus root peeled, sliced thin, then cut into quarters (optional)

1 cup carrots peeled, unless organic, and cut into thin matchsticks

Pinch of sea salt

Shoyu

1 teaspoon grated ginger juice to taste (optional)

Instructions

1. Heat oil in a skillet over medium flame and sauté the burdock with a pinch of sea salt for several minutes.

2. Add the lotus root and sauté for 3 more minutes.

3. Layer carrots on top and add water until the vegetables are almost covered.

4. Bring to a boil, then cover pan and simmer for 20 to 25 minutes until the vegetables are tender and the water is mostly absorbed. Add water during cooking if necessary.

5. Add a few drops of shoyu, gently mix, and cook for 5 more minutes.

6. Uncover and cook until any remaining water is almost gone.

7. Turn off flame, add ginger juice, and mix.

Variations: Use different combinations of one or more vegetables, such as onions, parsnips, or rutabagas. Use a pinch or two more sea salt or tamari instead of shoyu.

Scrambled Tofu

Light and tasty. Use vegetables you have on hand to create a delicious dish. Serve warm.

Serves 3 to 4

Ingredients

½ pound extra-firm tofu

½ to 1 tablespoon sesame or olive oil

2 to 3 cups vegetables (finely chopped or sliced red or yellow onions, broccoli, carrots, mushrooms, kale, zucchini, asparagus, etc)

½ to 1 teaspoon minced ginger

Scallions or fresh herbs (optional)

A pinch to ¼ teaspoon sea salt to taste

A few drops to ¼ teaspoon shoyu to taste

Turmeric or other seasonings to taste

Prepare the Tofu

1. Remove from package and rinse. If not using the whole package place the unused piece in a bowl with water, cover, and refrigerate.

2. Cut into several slices and press between two plates or paper towels for a few minutes to remove excess liquid.

3. Heat oil in a skillet on medium heat and fry tofu for several minutes on each side.

4. Remove tofu and cut into cubes

To Make the Tofu Scramble

1. Reheat skillet adding more oil if necessary and sauté onions and minced ginger until onions turn light brown. Add other vegetables and continue to cook until the vegetables are somewhat soft, adding water if necessary.

2. Add tofu and scallions and fresh herbs if using them and cook for two to three minutes longer.

3. Add salt, shoyu, and spices, and cook for another few minutes.

   Tip: Serve with a grain, quinoa, or steamed sourdough bread.

Variations: Use different vegetable combinations and seasonings.

Steamed Sourdough Bread Sandwich

This quick and delicious alternative to peanut butter and jelly is great for breakfast or to take with you for a mid-morning snack. Steaming the bread makes it more digestible.

Serves 1

Ingredients

One or two slices of fresh or frozen unyeasted whole wheat sourdough bread

Organic tahini

Naturally fermented organic sauerkraut

Instructions

1. Using a steamer pot or a regular pot with a steamer basket inside, add an inch or so of water to the pot, cover, and bring to a boil.

2. When the pot is producing steam, place the bread in the steamer for a minute or so and remove before it becomes too moist. If the bread is frozen it will take a little longer before it's soft and slightly moist. Steaming the bread helps to reconstitute it if it has become dry.

3. Spread a layer of tahini on the bread.

4. Add a little sauerkraut. This helps to balance the oil in the tahini and adds a salty flavor.

Variations: Use different varieties of unyeasted sourdough bread or different toppings, such as peanut butter, hummus, sliced avocado, or guacamole.

Stewed Tree Fruit

A quick and delicious dessert especially when tree fruits are in season. Serve warm.

Serves 3 to 4

Ingredients

½ cup apple juice

2 large apples, pears, or peaches rinsed and with the skin peeled if they're not organic

Small pinch of sea salt

Seasonings: sprinkle of cinnamon, ½ teaspoon minced ginger (optional)

Instructions

1. Cut or slice the fruit and place in pot.

2. Add apple juice, salt, and seasonings, if using.

3. Cover, bring to a boil, and simmer for 5 minutes.

4. Stir gently and continue to simmer with cover on for several minutes more until fruit becomes soft. Add more liquid if needed.

Variations: Use water instead of apple juice or a combination of apple juice and water. Add chopped pecans or other toppings.

Vegetable Stew Nishime Style

Long-cooked vegetable dishes are more warming and strengthening than raw or lightly cooked dishes. Each has a role in a plant-based diet. Nishime-style vegetable stews are considered long-cooked vegetable dishes and are based on traditional Japanese home cooking. They're prepared with round or root vegetables that are cooked in a heavy pot with just enough water to allow them to cook without losing their flavor. When prepared with sweet vegetables, such as onions, carrots, cabbage, and winter squash, they provide a natural sweet flavor to meals. I often prepare enough to last several days, sometimes eating it as a snack. Serve warm. Note: Leftovers can be eaten at room temperature or reheated in a steamer.

Serves 3 to 4

Essential Cookware

- 1½- or 2-quart heavy pot with tight-fitting lid. The vegetables will cook better when they almost fill the pot.

Ingredients

1 cup cabbage cut into chunks

1 cup winter squash cut into chunks

1 cup carrots roll-cut into large pieces

1-square-inch piece of kombu (kelp)

Small pinch of sea salt

Instructions

1. Rinse the kombu (kelp) and place on the bottom of the pot.

2. Add cabbage.

3. Add water so it covers the bottom of the pot by about a little more than ¼ inch or so. The amount of water needed so that there is practically none left at the end of cooking depends on the pot, the moisture in the vegetables, and their size.

4. Add winter squash.

5. Add carrots.

6. Add salt and bring to a boil.

7. Lower heat and simmer for 20 to 30 minutes until vegetables are tender.

   Tip: The vegetables will be sweeter when cooked without excess water, however, it takes experience with your stove, pot, and the moisture in the vegetables to gauge the amount of water needed until the vegetable are cooked through. It helps to check the pot several times and add a little water if necessary.

Variations: Use different combinations of one or more vegetables, such as onions, leeks, daikon radish, parsnips, or turnips. Add a little shoyu at the end, mix, and cook for several more minutes.

RESOURCES

FOOD PRODUCTS

Many of the food products I use are available at Whole Foods Market or other markets, at natural foods stores, and, in season, at farmers' markets. I shop online for those that aren't available locally.

Eden Foods. A large producer and distributor of natural foods, including traditional Japanese foods that are part of the macrobiotic diet. Located in Clinton, MI. www.edenfoods.com

Goldmine Natural Foods. Carries a large selection of high-quality traditional Japanese foods that are part of the macrobiotic diet. Located in Poway, CA. www.goldminenaturalfoods.com

Lundberg Family Farms. Grows and sells rice products, including organic brown rice. Lundberg publishes annual information about the arsenic content of their brown rice. Arsenic, a naturally occurring element, is found in some foods and in water. Because brown rice retains the nutritious outer layers of the rice kernel, it contains more arsenic than white rice does. Results of Lundberg's testing always fall well within the guidelines set by the FDA and other agencies. Soaking brown rice overnight in water, which I do to improve its digestibility, also removes some of the arsenic. www.lundberg.com

Maine Coast Sea Vegetables. Specializes in sustainably harvested seaweeds from the North Atlantic. Located in Hancock, ME. www.seaveg.com

Maine Seaweed. A family-owned farm that hand-harvests and dries Atlantic seaweeds. Located in Steuben, ME. www.theseaweedman.com

Natural Import Company. Carries a large selection of high-quality traditional Japanese natural foods that are part of the macrobiotic diet. Located in Rutherfordton, NC. www.naturalimport.com

Purcell Mountain Farms. Carries a large selection of beans, grains, and other plant-based food. Located in Moyie Springs, ID. www.purcellmountainfarms.com

Rhapsody Natural Foods. Produces organic tempeh, natto, and other products that are part of the macrobiotic diet. Located in Cabot, VT. www.rhapsodynaturalfoods.com

SiSalt. Produces high-quality naturally dried sea salt. www.sisalt.com

South River Miso. Produces organic miso using traditional methods. Located in Conway, MA. www.southrivermiso.com

ALEXANDER TECHNIQUE EDUCATION

For further information about the Alexander Technique or to find an Alexander Technique teacher, see the American Society for the Alexander Technique website: www.amsatonline.org

MACROBIOTIC PLANT-BASED DIET EDUCATION

The Strengthening Health Institute. Founded by Denny and Susan Waxman. Offers on-site courses, online courses, and health consultations. Located in Philadelphia, PA. www.shimacrobiotics.org

Macrobiotics of New England. Founded by Warren Kramer. Offers cooking instruction and health consultations. Located in Brighton, MA. www.macrobioticsnewengland.com

Great Life Global. Founded by Lino and Jane Stanchich. Offers educational programs and health consultations. Located in Asheville, NC. www.greatlifeglobal.com

BIBLIOGRAPHY

CHAPTER 1: ALLERGIES

Gross, Michael, Why did evolution give us allergies? www.cell.com, Current Biology, Volume 25, Issue 2, R53–55, 19 January 2015.

Meadows, Susannah, *The Other Side of Impossible: Ordinary People Who Faced Daunting Medical Challenges and Refused to Give Up* (Random House, 2017).

Sonnenburg, Justin, and Erica Sonnenburg, *The Good Gut: Taking Control of Your Weight, Your Mood, and Your Long-term Health* (Penguin Books, 2016).

CHAPTER 2: DIET AND HEALTH

Dufty, William, *Sugar Blues* (Grand Central Life & Style, 1986).

Ferré, Carl, *Acid Alkaline Companion: An Accompaniment to Herman Aihara's Acid and Alkaline* (George Ohsawa Macrobiotic Foundation, 2009).

Ferré, Julia, *Basic Macrobiotic Cooking, 20th Anniversary Edition: Procedures of Grain and Vegetable Cookery* (George Ohsawa Macrobiotic Foundation, 2007). One of my go-to books for cooking grains and beans.

Jack, Alex, and Sachi Kato, *One Peaceful World Cookbook,* (BenBella Books, 2017). Wonderful recipes with beautiful photographs.

Kushi, Michio, *Standard Macrobiotic Diet,* revised edition (One Peaceful World Press, 1996). Out-of-print, but used copies are available.

Kushi, Michio, and Alex Jack, *The Macrobiotic Path to Total Health: A Complete Guide to Naturally Preventing and Relieving More Than 200 Chronic Conditions and Disorders* (Ballantine Books, 2004).

Miyagi, Masao, and Evelyne Miyaji, *The ABCs of Vegan Home Cooking* (2014, available as a pdf download or formatted for Ebook or Apple iPad at blurb.com). A cookbook from the proprietors of Masao's Kitchen restaurant in Waltham, MA that's filled with useful information about cooking and recipes, including recipes for the delicious food served at Masao's Kitchen.

Silverstone, Alicia, *The Kind Diet: A Simple Guide to Feeling Great, Losing Weight, and Saving the Planet* (Rodale Books, 2009).

Waxman, Denny, *The Complete Macrobiotic Diet: 7 Steps to Feel Fabulous, Look Vibrant, and Think Clearly* (Pegasus Books, 2015). Reflects Denny Waxman's more than forty years of teaching. Has an excellent food section with recipes.

Macrobiotic Philosophy

Kushi, Michio, *The Book of Macrobiotics: The Universal Way of Health, Happiness & Peace,* revised edition (Square One, 2012).

Ohsawa, George, *Essential Ohsawa: From Food to Health, Happiness to Freedom* (George Ohsawa Macrobiotic Foundation, 2013).

Visual Diagnosis

Kushi, Michio, *Your Body Never Lies: The Complete Book of Oriental Diagnosis* (Square One, 2006).

Ohashi, Wataru, and Tom Monte, *Reading the Body: Ohashi's Book of Oriental Diagnosis* (Penguin Books, 1991).

CHAPTER 3: MANAGEMENT TECHNIQUES

Bullen, Christine V, and John F. Rockart, "A Primer on Critical Success Factors," Sloan School of Management Working Paper 1220–81, 1981; available at dspace.mit.edu/handle/ 1721.1/1988.

Dorfman, H. A., *Coaching the Mental Game* (Lyons Press, 2017). Presents leadership philosophies and strategies for peak performance in sports and everyday life.

Godin, Lisa, "Implementation Success—Critical Success Factors," IBM blog post, 2009, available at https://www.ibm.com/blogs/ watson-customer-engagement/2009/12/09/implementation-success-critical-success-factors/

Rockart, John F., "Chief Executives Define Their Own Data Needs," *Harvard Business Review,* March 1979.

CHAPTER 4: STAYING HEALTHY BEYOND DIET

Alexander, F. M., *The Use of the Self* (Orion, 2001).

Langer, Ellen, "Mindfulness in the Age of Complexity," *Harvard Business Review,* March 2014.

Ohashi, Wataru, *Do-It-Yourself Shiatsu: How to Perform the Ancient Japanese Art of Acupressure* (Penguin Books, 2001).

ACKNOWLEDGMENTS

I am deeply grateful to my family, friends, teachers, and colleagues for their love and support and for helping me bring this book to fruition.

Two years ago, after having worked on the book sporadically, I was ready to finish it. Six weeks later, I sent a rough draft to Phyllis Nahman for advice on how to proceed. Phyllis, a former English professor and friend who is familiar with plant-based diets, gave the draft a thumbs-up and encouraged me to continue. Several months later, I had a working draft, although it was far from a finished manuscript. I had always worked with teams, and I needed one now to make the book a reality.

First, I needed an editor. I am indebted to Kathy Carroll, my wonderful editor, for her patience and guidance. She has been unfailingly helpful and a relentless advocate for readers, asking thoughtful questions and making recommendations on their behalf.

One can't ask for a more supportive and caring friend and neighbor than Ellen Bick. She encouraged me and offered helpful advice whenever I needed it. Nancy Nitikman, a friend from my early days at Interactive Data Corporation, is a difference-maker. Nancy, who has many ties to the world of books, introduced me to Kathy Carroll and to others who provided helpful information. Ellen and Nancy, among other friends and neighbors, were always willing to review sections of the book and offer feedback.

A special thanks to Debra Byer, a chiropractor I've known for many years, who is familiar with the topics discussed in the book. When I needed feedback on the content, Debra graciously offered to review it. Larry Cohen, a neighbor with extensive knowledge of the many aspects of book publishing, was a great source of information. Larry kindly agreed to assist with the bibliography and lend his proofreading and copy-editing expertise when needed.

Thank you to Ruth Kilroy, Larry Anam, Russ Gilfus, and Eugene Silva, for their interest in this project and their timely advice.

My deepest thanks and appreciation also to people in my life whose guidance and example gave me the confidence to pursue my interests:

To my parents, Marion and Martin, who taught me the value of hard work and encouraged me to be independent. I am grateful to my father for fostering my enthusiasm for math, which led to my computer career.

To my grandparents, my great-aunt Sadie, and my extended family of aunts, uncles, and others who believed in me and were always there for me.

To the Golubs—my sister Pam, brother-in-law Jon, niece

Rachel, and nephews Adam and Steve—for supporting and even encouraging my dietary explorations.

To Jack Arnow and Frank Belvin, founders of Interactive Data, where I developed my systems and management skills, and to my many dedicated colleagues from whom I learned so much.

To Michio and Aveline Kushi and my macrobiotic friends and teachers, especially Denny and Susan Waxman, Warren and Fatim Kramer, and Leslie Frodema. Without the groundbreaking work of Michio and Aveline Kushi and the continued efforts of others, this book would not have been possible.

INDEX

ABOUT THE AUTHOR

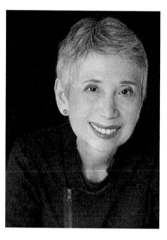

Ellen Wax has pursued extensive study with prominent leaders in their fields to deepen her understanding of natural health practices. A former Director of Systems Technology at Interactive Data Corporation, Ellen's career designing and managing mainframe computer operating systems spanned more than three decades and led to her interest in the application of management techniques from the workplace to complex problems in everyday life.